A GUIDE TO ARTHRITIS HOME HEALTH CARE

A GUIDE TO ARTHRITIS HOME HEALTH CARE

Edited by
JUDITH K. SANDS, R.N., ED.D.

Assistant Professor
School of Nursing
University of Virginia
Charlottesville, Virginia

Consultant
JUDITH H. MATTHEWS, R.N., M.S.N.

Director, Community Home Health Care
Waynesboro Community Hospital
Waynesboro, Virginia

WILEY

A Wiley-Medical Publication
JOHN WILEY & SONS
New York / Chichester / Brisbane / Toronto / Singapore

Library of Congress Cataloging-in-Publication Data

A Guide to arthritis home health care / edited by Judith K. Sands;
    consultant, Judith H. Matthews.
        p.   cm. — (A Wiley medical publication)
    Includes bibliographies and index.
        ISBN 0-471-63535-9 (pbk.)
        1. Arthritics—Home care. 2. Arthritis—Nursing.   I. Sands,
    Judith K. II. Matthews, Judith H.   III. Series.
        [DNLM: 1. Arthritis—nursing.   2. Home Care Services. WY 157.6
    G946]
    RC933.G85 1988
    649'.8—dc19
DNLM/DLC
for Library of Congress   88-5701
                                                                        CIP

Printed in the United States of America
10 9 8 7 6 5 4 3 2 1

*To my parents for always being there
and believing in me.
To Eric and David for the love
they bring to every day.*

Contributors

Susan E. Brunk, R.N., M.S.N., Health Educator, University of Virginia School of Nursing, Charlottesville, Virginia

Ann S. Goodson, R.N., B.S., Arthritis Clinic, University of Virginia Medical Center, Charlottesville, Virginia

Sarah A. Liddle, M.S., Administrator, Board for Rights of the Disabled, Commonwealth of Virginia, Richmond, Virginia

Judith K. Sands, R.N., Ed.D., Assistant Professor, School of Nursing, University of Virginia, Charlottesville, Virginia

Cynthia Stabenow Kulp, M.S., O.T.R., Coordinator, Arthritis Rehabilitation Unit, University of Virginia Medical Center, Charlottesville, Virginia

Trina Vecchiolla, R.N., M.S.N., Clinical Coordinator, Immobility, University of Virginia Medical Center, Charlottesville, Virginia

Stephen T. Wegener, Ph.D., Rehabilitation Research and Training Center, University of Virginia Medical Center, Charlottesville, Virginia

Preface

This book is an outgrowth of work supported by a grant from the National Institute on Disability and Rehabilitation Research, which established a Rehabilitation Research and Training Center in Arthritis and Low Back Pain at the University of Virginia Medical Center. As a subcomponent of one of the grant training projects, a series of workshops on arthritis home care was developed and offered to groups of public health nurses throughout Virginia. The response was enthusiastic. These nurses felt that this information about the nursing care of persons with arthritis needed to be formalized and added to the nursing literature. Their feedback served as the impetus for the development of this book.

Arthritis is a major national health problem affecting millions of individuals who are rarely seen in tertiary care inpatient settings. *A Guide to Arthritis Home Health Care* is designed to serve as a guide to the delivery of nursing care to arthritis patients in the home setting. Nursing includes multiple strategies that may be employed to improve an arthritis patient's comfort and positive adaptation to the disease. This book uses a multidisciplinary perspective but presents only those strategies that can be used safely and independently by nurses in the community. It is intended primarily to serve as a resource for practicing community health nurses, but it can also be used as a resource by nursing students at all levels who are studying the problems and needs of arthritis patients.

The content of the book is presented in a practical and applied rather than highly theoretical style. It is accompanied by multiple tools for assessment, planning, and patient teaching that can be adapted by readers for use in their own practice. A nursing process approach is used throughout the book. Case studies are included to assist the reader to review and apply the chapter content, and each chapter is accompanied by examples of patient resources that are available in the area, as well as information about where they can be acquired. No attempt has been made to deal with general approaches to community health nursing. The content is specific to the management of arthritis.

Chapters 1 and 2 discuss arthritis as a disease process and the drugs that may be used in treatment. The Pigg-Driscoll patient problems model (Pigg, Driscoll, & Caniff, 1985) is used to organize the remainder of the content. Chapters on mobility, daily living skills, and sexuality are included in Part 2, "Functional Alterations." Part 3, "Comfort Alterations," includes chapters on pain management, fatigue, and sleep disturbances. A chapter on psychologic and behavioral problems comprises Part 4, "Adaptation Alterations." Finally, Part 5, "Physical Alterations," contains chapters on total joint replacement and nutrition. It is the hope of the authors that this book will be a valuable and practical resource to guide nurses in delivering care to persons with arthritis.

JUDITH K. SANDS

Acknowledgments

Thanks and appreciation need to be expressed to many individuals who provided tangible and intangible assistance in the development of this book. First of all, enormous appreciation is expressed to Gwen Christmas and Jan Roy for their cheerful and patient work in typing and retyping the manuscript. Appreciation is also expressed to Lynn Kidder for her wonderful work with the illustrations. I also wish to acknowledge gratefully the careful and detailed content critique provided by Dr. Carolyn Brunner and the input of Judy Matthews and her staff at Waynesboro Community Hospital's Department of Community Home Health Care, who served as consultants to the book. The ongoing support of colleagues at the School of Nursing and the efforts of the editorial staff at John Wiley & Sons are also acknowledged. The Support of U.S. Department of Education NIDRR Grant No. G-0083-000-43 is acknowledged as the stimulus for the entire project.

I also wish to acknowledge the enthusiasm and babysitting provided by my parents and the tolerance of my children, which allowed me to complete another project successfully.

JUDITH K. SANDS

Contents

A GUIDE TO
ARTHRITIS
HOME HEALTH
CARE

PART 1

INCIDENCE AND TREATMENT OF ARTHRITIS

1

Arthritis and Its Treatment

Susan E. Brunk
Judith K. Sands

During the 1980s the Arthritis Foundation initiated a major advertising campaign that urged Americans to begin to "take arthritis seriously," and it is obvious that the astonishing prevalence statistics for the disease fully support this challenge. Statistics from the Arthritis Foundation indicate that arthritis affects more than 36 million Americans, or approximately one in seven (Rodnan, Schumacher, and Zvaifler, 1983). It extracts a financial toll of billions of dollars annually in physician payments, medication costs, and lost income. Arthritis is no respecter of age and afflicts individuals at any point along the life span, although the incidence statistics are heavily skewed toward the elderly. Its effects on an individual can range from mildly annoying to crippling and disabling.

Great progress has been made in recent years in our understanding and treatment of arthritis. The term *cure* is not applicable to arthritis at this time, but specialized research and treatment centers throughout the country have made significant gains in controlling the disease, preventing deformity and disability outcomes, and improving the general quality of life of individuals with arthritis.

Arthritis is a community health problem. Arthritis patients are not commonly hospitalized, except during acute disease exacerbations or for surgical interventions that attempt to control pain or improve mobility. Many patients simply manage their arthritis at home by themselves, consulting their family physician during periods of increased disease activity. Rheumatology specialists and multidisciplinary care centers treat only a minority of the nation's arthritis patients. Therefore, millions of patients with mild or moderate disease may have only minimal exposure to the treatment approaches being developed and tested in arthritis research centers. The Arthritis Foundation attempts to bridge this gap with its massive public and patient education efforts. Their numerous publications emphasize responsible self-care management for arthritis patients. Still, it is apparent that many individuals are not reached by these approaches.

The community health nurse is an excellent potential source of information concerning arthritis treatment and home management. Community health nurses may organize and offer community education programs about arthritis management. They may also provide or supervise needed care in the home. Given the current status of our health care reimbursement programs, opportunities for home care are usually limited to new diagnoses, episodes of disease exacerbation, and needed care for rehabilitation following surgery. Ongoing support for chronic arthritis is rarely financially possible. But even within these limitations, the uniqueness of the home environment provides the nurse with the opportunity to intervene successfully in multiple aspects of the patient's living situation in order to modify or minimize the negative effects of the disease process. Even when arthritis is not the primary problem for which the family is being visited, its effects can seriously limit the successful functioning of the entire family. In these situations, successful interventions for the family member with arthritis can make indirect but important contributions to improving the quality of life of the entire family. This holistic approach to family care planning is particularly important when the family member with arthritis also assumes the role of caretaker for the nurse's assigned patient.

Community health nurses, especially in rural areas, may function independently, without the benefit of extensive backup and support from other interdisciplinary professionals. They may be requested to implement and monitor drug protocols such as the administration of gold under the treatment guidelines of physicians from a referral arthritis treatment center. It is therefore essential that these nurses be knowledgeable about a wide variety of treatment modalities for arthritis and skillful in assessing situations in which these modalities can be effectively implemented. The subsequent chapters of this book provide the necessary knowledge base for the nurse to intervene safely and appropriately in a patient's home setting in order to improve the patient's adaptation to the multiple challenges of arthritis. The remainder of this chapter provides a foundation for understanding the various disease processes of arthritis and their medical and nursing management.

THE NORMAL JOINT

The joints of the body are classified into three major categories reflecting their relative degree of movement and the type of tissue present in the joint. Fibrous or synarthrotic joints are immovable joints in which the bone surfaces come in direct contact with each other and are fastened together by fibrous tissue, cartilage, or bone. Fibrous joints are found along the suture lines of the bones of the skull. Cartilaginous or amphiarthrotic joints comprise the second category. They are slightly movable joints connected by cartilage. The symphysis pubis of the pelvis and the bodies of the spinal vertebrae that are joined by intervertebral discs are examples of cartilaginous joints. The third category consists of the synovial or diarthrodial joints. Although these joints are classified as freely movable, their actual degree of movement varies from almost none to movement in many planes.

In a synovial joint, the articulating ends of the bones are not connected directly but are indirectly linked by a strong fibrous joint capsule. The bony surfaces are covered with thin layers of articular cartilage that slide past each other during movement. These are the joints most commonly affected by arthritis. The subcategories of synovial joints are organized according to the different movement axes involved. Common examples include the gliding joints of the hands and feet; the hinge joints of the elbows and fingers; the condylar joints of the knees; and the ball-and-socket joints of the shoulders and hips.

Figure 1-1 illustrates the basic structure of the diarthrodial joint. The actual joint is enclosed in a capsule whose outer layers are composed of dense fibrous tissue that gradually merges with the periosteum, the membrane that covers the bone. The inside of the joint capsule is lined with the synovium, a membrane that forms a very thin lining, usually only a few cells thick. The two bone ends are covered by a smooth layer of cartilage that forms a cushion and acts as a shock absorber during weight bearing and joint motion. The cartilage compresses when force is applied and expands when pressure is released. The synovium folds around the margins of the articulating surface of the cartilage but does not actually cover it. It does, however, cover the tendons that pass through the joint, as well as the free margins of other intra-articular structures such as ligaments. These synovial folds allow a significant amount of joint stretching to occur without producing tissue damage.

The synovial membrane produces the slippery synovial fluid that fills the small space around and between the ends of the two bones. It keeps the joint well lubricated for easy movement. In the adult, the cartilage has no direct blood supply, lymphatic channels, or nerve endings. It depends on the synovial fluid for both nourishment and waste removal. The synovial fluid itself is nourished by a rich network of capillaries that are concentrated in the synovium directly adjacent to the joint cavity, thus facilitating rapid diffusion. There is normally no more than 2–3 cc of synovial fluid in a joint space the size of the knee.

Outside the joint capsule are muscles, tendons, and ligaments that

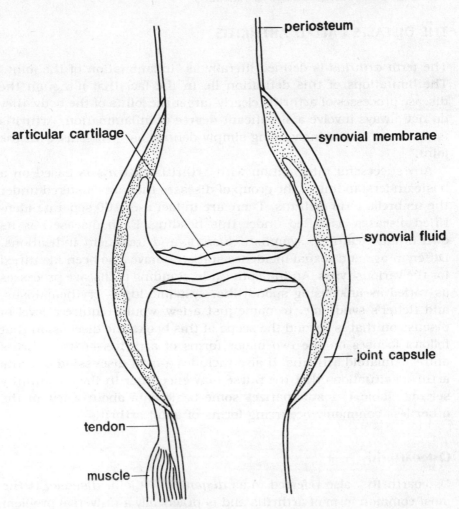

Figure 1–1. The diarthrodial, synovial joint.

provide support and stability to the joint and assist in movement. The tendons attach the muscles to bones, and the ligaments connect the bones to each other. Fluid-filled sacs called *bursae* are distributed among the various joint structures to assist them in moving smoothly against each other. The entire synovial joint structure is highly efficient and has such a low level of friction that the articular cartilage only rarely must endure significant stresses. But any factor that interferes with the articulating surface, the process of synovial nourishment, or the natural neuromuscular shock-absorbing properties can produce abrupt or gradual breakdown in joint function.

THE DISEASES CALLED ARTHRITIS

The term *arthritis* is defined literally as "inflammation of the joint." The limitations of this definition lie in the fact that although the disease processes of arthritis clearly target the joints of the body, they do not always involve a significant degree of inflammation. Arthritis is therefore increasingly being simply defined as "problems with the joint."

Any successful intervention with arthritis patients is based on a basic understanding of the group of diseases that are clustered under the umbrella term *arthritis*. There are in fact over 100 separate identified diseases classified under this heading. Each disease has its own unique features, symptom clusters, and treatment indications. Different age and sexual incidence statistics have also been identified for the various types. An in-depth understanding of disease processes as varied as ankylosing spondylitis, systemic lupus erythematosus, and Reiter's syndrome, to name just a few, would require a level of discussion that is beyond the scope of this book. The discussion that follows focuses on the two major forms of arthritis—osteoarthritis and rheumatoid arthritis. It also includes a brief discussion of acute arthritis situations that the nurse may encounter in the community setting. Table 1–1 summarizes some basic data about a few of the other less commonly occurring forms of adult arthritis.

Osteoarthritis

Osteoarthritis, also referred to as *degenerative joint disease*, is the most common form of arthritis and is practically a universal problem in the aging adult population. Virtually 100% of the over-65 population show some evidence of the disease on x-ray film even if they are clinically asymptomatic. It is a chronic disease of unknown etiology that can be mild or lead to significant pain and disability, especially when the involved joints are critical to the activities of daily living.

Osteoarthritis may be classified as primary or secondary. Primary osteoarthritis is idiopathic and occurs without an obvious reason. It occurs widely in the aging population and affects women more frequently than men. Secondary arthritis develops from an identifiable cause such as fracture, cartilage or ligament trauma, or congenital or metabolic alterations in the cartilage. It can occur at virtually any age and in any joint.

Table 1-1 Characteristics of Selected Forms of Arthritis

Disease	Age at Onset	Sex Ratio	Description	Treatment
Systemic lupus erythematosus	Highest incidence during late adolescence and early adulthood.	A 6:1 female:male ratio.	Chronic inflammatory disease that may affect many different organs. Onset is variable, and course follows pattern of exacerbation and remission. Wide variety of symptoms: characteristic butterfly facial rash, fatigue, weakness, and polyarthritis are common.	Aspirin in antiinflammatory doses. Corticosteroid therapy. Supportive care.
Polymyositis	Any age.	A 2:1 female:male ratio.	An inflammatory disorder of striated muscle that causes symmetric weakness and some atrophy. Onset and progression are highly variable. Symptoms include proximal muscle weakness and skin rash.	Corticosteroid therapy, supportive care, physical and occupational therapy.

Table 1-1   Characteristics of Selected Forms of Arthritis (*Cont.*)

Disease	Age at Onset	Sex Ratio	Description	Treatment
Ankylosing spondylitis	Late adolescence to middle adulthood.	Males affected more often than females, and disease is usually more severe.	A chronic inflammatory disease that initially affects the lower back and thoracic spine. It may follow an ascending pattern, affecting the joints between the ribs and vertebrae. Symptoms are initially mild (pain and stiffness in the lower back) but may progress, limiting back flexion and chest expansion.	Nonsteroidal anti-inflammatory drug therapy. Physical therapy and exercise to prevent deformity and maintain adequate lung expansion.

| Reiter's syndrome | Young adult years. | Predominantly affects males; rare in females. | An acute inflammatory syndrome that begins with urethritis, usually sexually acquired, and is followed by the development of conjunctivitis (usually mild) and arthritis. The onset of arthritis is acute and typically affects the weight-bearing joints. Involved joints are acutely inflamed. Complete recovery is typical, but recurrences are common. | Essentially symptomatic. Nonsteroidal anti-inflammatory drugs. Temporary bed rest with splinting may be needed. |

Pathology

The disease process of osteoarthritis involves the gradual breakdown of articular cartilage and the exposure of the underlying bone. Inflammation is not generally a major component of the disease process, although secondary synovitis can play a role. The articular surface fissures and splits in the superficial layers at specific sites that gradually merge and deepen until relatively large areas of bare bone surface are created. The cause of the initial cartilage change is not completely understood, although chronic or acute trauma is suspected to play a role. Once the cellular changes are initiated, simple mechanical factors appear to play a major role in the ongoing cartilage destruction. In addition to the cartilaginous destruction, osteophyte spur formation occurs at the joint margins. Bone spurs and bone cysts develop in the affected joints as the disease progresses.

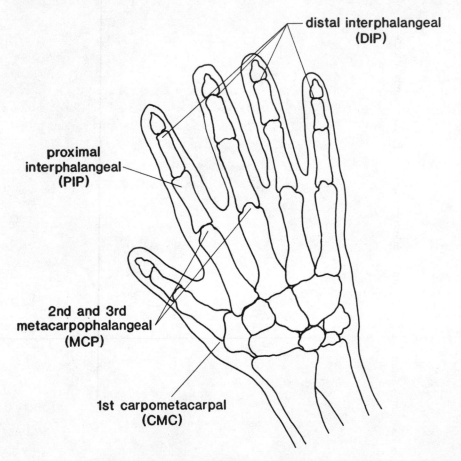

Figure 1–2. Joints of the hands.

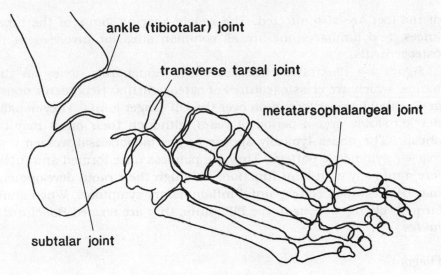

ankle (tibiotalar) joint

transverse tarsal joint

metatarsophalangeal joint

subtalar joint

Figure 1–3. Joints of the feet.

Synovitis may be triggered by the release of cartilage crystals that stimulate inflammation.

Figures 1-2 and 1-3 illustrate the joints of the hands and feet. Osteoarthritis typically affects the proximal and distal interphalangeal (PIP and DIP) joints of the fingers and the first carpometacarpal (CMC) joints of the hand. The first metatarsophalangeal (MTP) joints

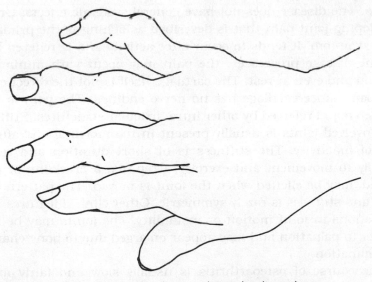

Figure 1–4. Heberden's and Bouchard's nodes.

of the foot are also affected. The weight-bearing joints of the hips, knees, and lumbar spine are all common sites for involvement in osteoarthritis.

Figure 1-4 illustrates Heberden's and Bouchard's nodes on the hands, which are classic features of osteoarthritis. Heberden's nodes are created by spur formation over the DIP finger joints. They usually develop slowly over a period of years, although their onset may be abrupt. The nodes typically appear in postmenopausal women and follow a symmetric pattern. They are painless once formed and interfere minimally with joint function, although their rapid development may be accompanied by painful inflammatory symptoms. When similar joint changes occur in the PIP joints, they are termed *Bouchard's nodes*.

Diagnosis

The diagnosis of osteoarthritis is usually established through a patient history and physical examination, combined with x-ray and laboratory findings that exclude other disease processes. X-ray films may appear normal if the pathologic changes are early or mild. There is usually a positive correlation between clinical symptoms and x-ray abnormalities, but the x-ray films may not accurately reflect the severity of the symptoms experienced by any particular patient.

Symptoms and Clinical Course

The signs and symptoms of osteoarthritis are usually localized to the joints. The disease does not have general systemic effects. Gradually developing joint pain that is described as aching is the primary disease symptom. It tends to occur after activity and is relieved by rest. As the disease progresses, the pain may occur with minimal joint motion and even at rest. The cartilage itself is not the direct cause of the pain, since cartilage has no nerve endings. The pain is instead triggered and referred by other intra-articular structures. Stiffness in the involved joints is usually present in the morning and after periods of inactivity. The stiffness is of short duration and responds rapidly to movement and exercise. Crepitus, a crackling or grating sound, may be elicited when the joint is moved. The pattern of joint pain and stiffness is rarely symmetric. Other clinical features include limitations in joint motion or instability. The joints may be slightly tender to palpation and may appear enlarged due to bony changes or inflammation.

The course of osteoarthritis is usually slow and fairly mild, although in some cases the process of joint degeneration can be abrupt and severe. Involvement of major weight-bearing joints and/or the spine appears to be associated with an increased incidence of disability and is a common indication for total joint replacement. Not all patients inevitably deteriorate, but neither is osteoarthritis always a benign disease.

Joint Deformities. Joint deformities are less common with osteoarthritis than with rheumatoid arthritis, but they can occur from the loss of cartilage and extensive bony overgrowth that lead to joint enlargement and malalignment. Genu valgum ("knock knees"), hallux valgus and hammertoes, and varied gait changes can all occur from joint destruction and instability.

Rheumatoid Arthritis

Rheumatoid arthritis is a chronic systemic inflammatory disease of unknown etiology. It is estimated to affect about 1–2% of the adult population. The usual onset of the disease is between the ages of 20 and 60, with a peak incidence between 35 and 40. Rheumatoid arthritis affects women more than men by a ratio of about 3:1, although the ratio is closer to 5:1 in the under-60 age group.

Although the cause of rheumatoid arthritis remains unknown, there is increasing evidence that immunologic factors play an important role. The disease is usually progressive, and follows a typical pattern of exacerbation and remission over many years. The disease pattern in any individual is both highly variable and unpredictable. It is difficult for patients and families to understand the disease process, and its lack of predictability can make it difficult for them to cope. Serious deformity is a possible outcome of rheumatoid arthritis when the process of joint inflammation is not interrupted, but it is not inevitable. Although a cure for the disease remains frustratingly elusive, comprehensive treatment programs have made enormous strides in controlling its effects. Even in its most virulent forms, the disease process tends to become less aggressive over time. Early treatment intervention is essential to prevent irreversible joint destruction.

Pathology

Rheumatoid arthritis is not simply localized in the joints, but the joint disease symptoms are by far its most characteristic feature. The joint disease is inflammatory, and the synovial membrane is the primary site of inflammation. The synovial membrane begins to proliferate in response to a poorly understood stimulus. The process is believed to be a disorder of immune system functioning, perhaps initiated by a combination of environmental and genetic factors. Most individuals with rheumatoid arthritis carry the rheumatoid factor in their blood. It is an antibody that is produced in response to one of the body's own immunoglobulins. Viral agents may alter the structure of the immunoglobulin slightly, and a genetic predisposition may increase the chance that the altered immunoglobulin will be perceived as foreign. When this occurs, an antigen–antibody reaction is started that results in the formation of immune complexes. Whether localized or circulating, these complexes generally activate the complement system and involve other reticuloendothelial cells in the inflammatory response. Released enzymes help to destroy the targeted antigen but may also destroy the body's own tissues. The inflammatory process causes increased blood flow to the joint and increased vascular permeability. These factors combine to produce the classic symptoms of joint warmth and swelling. Palpation of the involved joints reveals boggy tissue, and excess fluid can be aspirated from the joint.

The characteristic joint damage of rheumatoid arthritis is due to two major processes. The first involves cartilage breakdown resulting from enzymes called *proteases* in the synovial fluid that cause a form of proteolytic digestion. The most destructive element, however, involves the formation of pannus, a vascular granulation tissue, which grows over the surface of the cartilage. In ongoing disease, the pannus forms adhesions and begins to adhere to opposing articular surfaces. This can result in fibrous ankylosis of the joint surfaces and eventually in bony ankylosis. Scarring, adhesions, and capsular shrinkage weaken and alter joint structures and limit joint mobility. When the joint changes of rheumatoid arthritis occur, the basic mechanical factors of weight bearing and muscle pull work directly against the joint and contribute to the development of the classic deformities of rheumatoid arthritis.

Congestion and synovial fluid accumulation contribute to the development of the *gel phenomenon*, which produces the classic symptom of stiffness of rheumatoid arthritis. The fluid appears to accumulate with rest and then must be slowly reabsorbed with muscle activity. The degree and persistence of gelling may assume clinical significance as an indirect measure of disease activity, since during acute flare-ups of rheumatoid arthritis the stiffness may persist throughout most of the day.

Diagnosis

The diagnosis of rheumatoid arthritis is easily made in the advanced stages of the disease but is not as easily established in the early stages. This is particularly true when the classic joint symptoms are not prominent or when only a single joint is initially involved. The symptoms experienced by the patient are important parts of the diagnostic process. The classic stiffness is present in the morning or after periods of inactivity and gradually eases as the individual moves about. In acute flare-ups, however, the stiffness may persist for hours or even all day. The degree of pain experienced is also variable and may not be directly related to the degree of inflammation present. It occurs primarily with joint movement and exercise.

Additional factors that support the diagnosis of rheumatoid arthritis include laboratory identification of the rheumatoid factor, synovial fluid analysis, and x-ray documentation of bone demineralization and erosion in affected joints. The rheumatoid factor is present in up to 70% of persons with rheumatoid arthritis, but it is not specific to this particular disease process. Moderate anemia of a normochromic, normocytic variety is another common laboratory finding in rheumatoid arthritis. It is associated with low serum iron levels and is quite resistant to iron therapy. The erythrocyte sedimentation rate tends to parallel the disease pattern and is elevated during periods of increased disease activity.

The diagnostic criteria proposed by the American Rheumatism Association are presented in Table 1–2. Classic rheumatoid arthritis is diagnosed when any combination of *seven* or more symptoms or findings is present in a patient with continuous disease for at least 6 weeks. A definite diagnosis requires the presence of at least *five* of the criteria.

Symptoms and Clinical Course

Pain, stiffness, swelling, redness, heat, and limitation of movement are all classic symptoms of rheumatoid arthritis, but they may not be the first symptoms experienced by the patient. Rheumatoid arthritis may begin with nonspecific symptoms such as fatigue, weakness, anorexia, and generalized aching. Actual joint symptoms slowly appear over a period of weeks or months. Patients may, however, experience an abrupt onset of acute polyarthritis that may be accompanied

Table 1–2   Criteria for the Classification of Rheumatoid Arthritis

A. Classic Rheumatoid Arthritis

This diagnosis requires seven of the following criteria. The joint signs or symptoms must be continuous for at least 6 weeks.

1. Morning stiffness
2. Pain on motion or tenderness of at least one joint
3. Swelling in at least one joint
4. Swelling of at least one other joint
5. Symmetric joint swelling with simultaneous involvement of the same joint on both sides of the body
6. Subcutaneous nodules
7. X-ray changes typical of rheumatoid arthritis
8. Presence of rheumatoid factor
9. Poor mucin precipitate from synovial fluid
10. Characteristic histologic changes in the synovium
11. Characteristic histologic changes in nodules

B. Definite Rheumatoid Arthritis

This diagnosis requires five of the above criteria. The joint signs or symptoms must be continuous for at least 6 weeks.

Source: Reprinted from the *Primer on the Rheumatic Diseases*, 8th edition, copyright 1983. Used by permission of the Arthritis Foundation.

by fever and other typical systemic signs of illness. The pattern of onset does not necessarily appear to be related to the eventual progress of the disease.

Rheumatoid arthritis can affect any diarthrodial joint of the body and in virtually any sequence, but the typical pattern of joint involvement is bilaterally symmetric and polyarticular. In its early stages the disease may present unilaterally or in just a single joint, although this is not common. The small joints of the hands, wrists, feet, and knees are early targets. As the disease progresses, the hips, ankles, shoulders, elbows, cervical spine, and mandibular joints may all become involved. Table 1–3 compares the major features of rheumatoid arthritis and osteoarthritis.

Systemic Symptoms. Although joint manifestations are the primary and characteristic features of rheumatoid arthritis, the disease also produces diverse systemic effects. Common patient complaints in-

Table 1–3   Comparison of Rheumatoid Arthritis and Osteoarthritis

Factor	Rheumatoid Arthritis	Osteoarthritis
Age at onset	Young and middle-aged	Middle aged and older
Sex ratio	Females:males, 3:1	Females:males, 2:1
Disease process	Inflammatory	Degenerative
Cause of disease	Unknown	Unknown
Nature of illness	Systemic symptoms	Local joint involvement only
Course of disease	Pattern of exacerbation and remission is common	Chronic, slowly progressive
Joints affected	PIPs, MCPs, MTPs, wrists, knees. Pattern is usually symmetric	DIPs, CMCs, weight-bearing joints, MTPs, knees, spine, hip. Pattern is usually asymmetric involving one or more joints
Systemic factors	Anemia, fatigue, subcutaneous nodules, low-grade fever, anorexia	Not usually present

clude generalized muscle aches, extreme fatigue, anorexia, weight loss, and episodes of low-grade fever. Specific extra-articular features such as subcutaneous nodules, lymph node enlargement, neuropathics, ocular effects, vasculitis, pericarditis, and pulmonary disease may also be a part of the overall disease process. Their presence is usually not clinically significant except in aggressive, rapidly developing disease states in which the systemic effects may become a prominent focus of treatment.

Subcutaneous nodules are the most common extra-articular symptom of rheumatoid arthritis. They occur in about 20% of all rheumatoid arthritis patients. The nodules are firm, nontender masses that form in the subcutaneous or deeper layers of the connective tissue. They may be very small or grow to several centimeters in size. They appear on the extensor surface of the forearm near the elbow, at the Achilles tendon, or at other sites that are routinely subjected to mechanical pressures. The nodules seldom cause pain or produce other symptoms, and they are not removed unless infection or skin breakdown occurs, since they typically regrow.

Lymph node enlargement can be another systemic feature of rheumatoid arthritis. The lymph nodes closest to the affected joints tend to be enlarged, but node involvement may be found in areas quite distant from the inflamed joints. Palpable splenomegaly is also present, which can lead to low white blood cell counts.

Rheumatoid arthritis does not typically affect the central nervous system, but abnormalities may be found in the peripheral nerves. Neurologic symptoms may also result from nerve compression. Carpal tunnel syndrome from medial nerve compression is a common cause of paresthesias in the hand. Patients experience burning pain, tingling, or numbness, particularly at night. Muscle weakness may develop as the condition worsens and may necessitate surgical release. Ulnar, radial, and tibial nerve involvement is also possible.

Sjögren's syndrome is present in about 10% of rheumatoid arthritis patients. Its primary symptoms are reduced lacrimal and salivary gland secretion, although any mucous membranes can be affected. Dryness in the eyes causes them to feel sandy or gritty. Dry mouth causes the patient to crave oral fluids. Symptomatic treatment is usually adequate. Artificial tears eyedrops, hard candy, and artificial saliva reduce the effects of dryness.

Other possible systemic disease effects include vasculitis, pericarditis, respiratory fibrosis, hematologic abnormalities, and ocular lesions. These manifestations may range from asymptomatic or mild to life-threatening. Treatment is usually symptom specific.

Joint Deformities. Progressive joint destruction that results in joint deformity is one of the most distressing potential outcomes of rheumatoid arthritis. The prevention of joint deformities is a significant ongoing care goal for arthritis patients, since a decrease in functional capacities and self-care abilities is an almost inevitable outcome of their development.

Problems with the joints of the hands are among the most common. As the disease progresses, the soft tissues become less firm and joint support less effective, so that even the normal pressures of daily use can cause deformities to develop. Figure 1-5 illustrates several of the classic deformities of the hands.

1. Ulnar deviation (Figure 1-5A)—subluxation or partial dislocation of the MCP joints due to muscle pulls on unstable joints. This deformity occurs frequently.

2. Swan neck deformity (Figure 1-5B)—the PIP joint is hyperextended while the DIP joint is in flexion. With this deformity, the individual loses the ability to flex and therefore cannot make a fist or hold small objects.

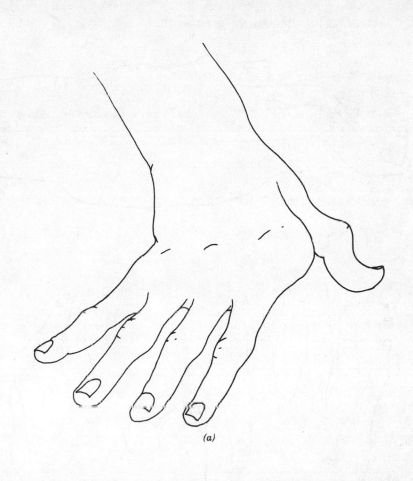

(a)

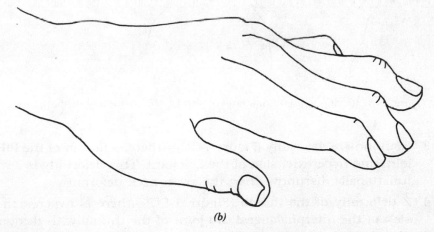

(b)

Figure 1-5. Classic rheumatoid arthritis deformitites of the hands: (a) ulnar deviation, (b) swan neck.

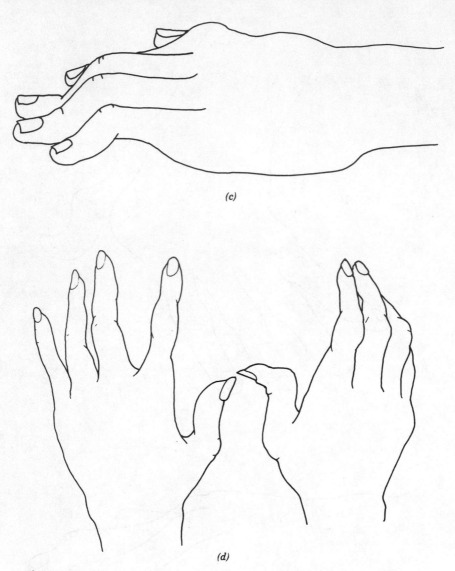

Figure 1–5. (Continued) (c) boutonniere, and (d) "Z" deformity of the thumb.

3. Boutonniere deformity (Figure 1-5C)—there is flexion of the PIP joint and hyperextension of the DIP joint. This deformity is less functionally disruptive than the swan neck deformity.
4. Z deformity of the thumb (Figure 1-5D)—there is hyperextension of the interphalangeal (IP) joint of the thumb with flexion of the MCP joint. This deformity compromises the individual's

ability to pinch and pick up small objects due to instability of the IP joint.

The most common joint deformities that occur in the feet are hallux valgus, in which the great toe is displaced toward the other toes, and hammertoes. Genu valgum or "knock knees" is another joint outcome of rheumatoid arthritis. Figure 1-6 illustrates the common deformities that may occur in the lower extremities.

The course of rheumatoid arthritis is highly variable and cannot be predicted with any degree of accuracy at the onset of the disease. Some patients experience an unrelenting worsening of their disease process, while others experience periods of acute exacerbation interspersed with relatively symptom free intervals. The presence of rheumatoid arthritis usually becomes more constant as time passes despite therapy. Only rarely is the actual disease process directly fatal, but its multiple effects on the body leave the individual with increased vulnerability to other diseases.

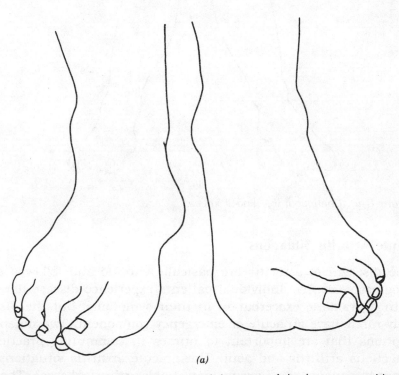

(a)

Figure 1–6. Common rheumatoid arthritis deformities of the lower extremities: (a) hallux valgus and hammertoes.

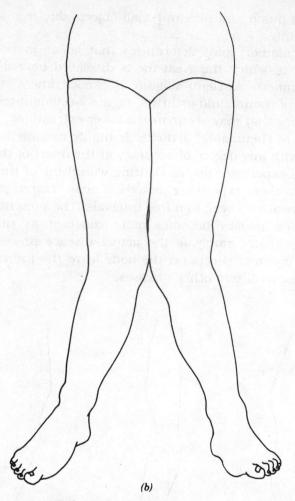

Figure 1–6. (Continued) (b) "knock knees."

Acute Arthritis Situations

The diseases of arthritis are basically chronic and follow a slowly progressive course. Individual patients experience disease flare-ups, with a dramatic exacerbation in their symptoms, but the diseases only rarely have an acute or emergency component. Two notable exceptions that are important to nurses in community practice are infectious arthritis and gout. These acute arthritis situations may occur in patients who have no identifiable arthritic disease. The community health nurse needs to be aware of the signs and symptoms of these disease processes, as well as the patients who may be at risk for developing them. Early identification and prompt referral for treatment can make an important difference in the patient's treatment response and comfort.

Infectious Arthritis

Infectious agents can cause arthritis through several different mechanisms. Direct penetration following traumatic injury is one method, but organisms can also trigger hypersensitivity and immunologically induced inflammation due to their presence elsewhere in the body. Since the synovial membrane is extremely vascular, microorganisms can also gain access to the membrane or synovial fluid directly from the blood. Infectious arthritis is also a rare but extremely serious complication of total joint replacement.

Direct invasion from the blood is the most common cause of infectious arthritis. Organisms become trapped in the joint and multiply rapidly. The invading organisms can be bacteria, viruses, or fungi. The nature of the specific organism largely determines the aggressiveness and speed of the disease process.

Susceptibility to infectious arthritis is not always clear, since it may complicate a known arthritis situation or be associated with another apparently unrelated medical condition. Anything that compromises immune system functioning, such as steroid use, increases the risk. Aging decreases immune function, and elderly patients are at risk for infectious arthritis after pneumonia and other systemic bacteremias. Previous injury of a joint also increases the risk. Total joint replacement patients need specific instructions about preventing bacterial infection, particularly in the urinary tract (see Chapter 8). A final high-risk group consists of young, sexually active individuals who may be exposed to or harbor unidentified gonococcal organisms.

Acute localized joint pain is the primary symptom of infectious arthritis. Redness, swelling, fever, and other systemic signs of infection may also be present. This symptom pattern is characteristic of gram-positive organisms. Infections caused by viruses and gram-negative organisms tend to produce migratory polyarthralgias, skin rashes, fever, and tenosynovitis.

A definitive diagnosis of infectious arthritis can be made only by successful culture of the organism. However, this is often not possible. Most viruses and some bacteria are rarely cultured successfully.

Staphylococcus aureus, Neisseria gonorrhoeae, and pneumococci are frequently encountered. Without organism growth on culture, the diagnosis is established by the patient's history, the symptoms, and the response to treatment.

Prompt treatment is important to prevent irreversible joint damage. The patient is often hospitalized to receive appropriate parenteral antibiotic therapy, joint immobilization, and pain control. With early identification and prompt treatment, complete recovery is usually possible.

Gout

Gout is characterized by acute attacks of arthritis that are caused by the deposition of uric acid crystals within the joint. It results from either overproduction or decreased excretion of uric acid through the kidneys. Primary gout results from genetic defects in purine metabolism, whereas secondary gout can occur as a sequela of a variety of conditions and medications.

Patients at risk for secondary gout include individuals with cancer, particularly those receiving chemotherapy. Hyperuricemia results from the rapid turnover of purines in the body. Renal insufficiency and failure result in decreased glomerular filtration of uric acid and can also cause gout. Medications such as penicillin, thiazide diuretics, and low-dose aspirin therapy interfere with the tubular secretion of uric acid, and steroid use increases the metabolism of purines in the body. All can produce secondary gout.

An attack of gout occurs when uric acid crystals precipitate within the joint, initiating an acute inflammatory response. A typical attack affects just one joint, often the first MTP joint of the foot. Acute pain and inflammation are the primary symptoms, and they may persist for days or weeks.

The diagnosis must be carefully established to rule out infectious arthritis. A definitive diagnosis is made when crystals are found in the joint fluid. Hyperuricemia alone is present in many individuals without symptoms of gout and is not diagnostic.

Treatment is aimed at reducing inflammation and controlling pain. Colchicine is the drug of choice, administered either orally or parenterally. Nonsteroidal anti-inflammatory drugs may be substituted if the patient experiences significant nausea, vomiting, or diarrhea. After the acute phase resolves, treatment will continue with either probenecid to increase uric acid excretion or allopurinol to block its production.

MEDICAL MANAGEMENT OF ARTHRITIS

Since neither rheumatoid arthritis nor osteoarthritis can be cured, the major focus of medical treatment is on the management of symptoms and the prevention of joint deformity and loss of function. Although rheumatoid arthritis and osteoarthritis are obviously very different disease processes, the overall treatment plans for both share many features. Despite its common characteristic symptoms, arthritis is experienced differently by virtually every patient. Arthritis challenges the care team to individualize the planned treatment regimen to meet the unique needs and responses of every patient.

One of the first hurdles to be overcome in establishing a treatment protocol is the widespread belief that little or nothing can be done for arthritis. It is important that patients know that although a cure for their disease is not possible, its effects can be significantly reduced or modified by treatment. Addressing this issue is an ongoing concern for all professionals involved with the patient's care. A comprehensive medical treatment plan usually includes appropriate medication prescriptions, pain control measures, a therapeutic exercise plan, joint protection measures, and the use of assistive devices as indicated. The overall plan also aims at balancing activity and rest; maintaining good nutrition; achieving and maintaining optimal body weight; and supporting the patient's efforts at effective adaptation to the stresses of chronic illness. In advanced disease, surgical interventions may also become an integral part of the total treatment plan.

Unproven remedies are commonly employed by patients with arthritis, running the gamut from copper bracelets and special diets to the dangerous, unsupervised use of high-dose steroids. Unproven remedies affect the overall arthritis treatment plan in a variety of ways. They may be used by the patient as an adjunct to the physician's regimen or in place of it. Traditionally, it has been difficult for health professionals to deal with unproven remedies. There is a strong tendency for professionals to disparage these approaches to disease management and to become annoyed with patients who use them. This attitude can result in the erection of a barrier between the health professional and the individual receiving care. It is important that all involved professionals proceed with sensitivity in this area, evaluating each remedy only from the perspective of potential harm or excessive cost. If the potential for harm exists, it is both legitimate and necessary to intervene. If the remedy is not potentially harmful, however, it is wise not to interfere with the patient's choice. Our understanding of psychophysiologic disease principles and placebos is not sophisticated or complete enough to explain all of the subjective claims of symptom improvement routinely reported by patients. Approaches to unproven remedies will be further discussed in Chapter 7 under the heading "Limitations in Insight."

Once the overall treatment plan has been established, its components remain in place for months or even years. Medication, exercise, rest, nutrition, and joint protection are lifelong needs for arthritis patients. The physician coordinator will, of course, adjust the various components of the plan as indicated over time by the patient's response and the clinical course. But once the parameters have been established, it is the community health nursing professional who will be called upon to assist the patient to adapt optimally to the limitations of the disease process and the restrictions of the treatment regimen in everyday life.

NURSING MANAGEMENT OF ARTHRITIS

The role of the professional nurse in the total treatment plan for arthritis is essential, especially in the community setting. While the physician and other interdisciplinary professionals establish the broad outlines of the overall treatment plan, it is usually the nurse who works with the patient and family in the home environment to implement it and make it successful. The strict limits on the number of reimbursable home visits make it imperative that the nurse maximize each contact with the patient and family. The community health nurse is often the only team member to see the patient in the home environment. This direct contact allows for an in-depth assessment of the patient's physical surroundings and family dynamics that is available to no one else. If treatment regimens are to work, they must be tailored to the unique strengths and limitations of the family's home setting. Community health nurses have always enjoyed a hard-won reputation for creativity in adapting medical regimens to the patient's unique home environment. Providing care to the arthritis patient again challenges that creativity.

Community health nursing focuses on assisting patients and their families to adapt successfully to the challenges and limitations imposed on their desired lifestyle by their illness. For arthritis patients these challenges are often extensive, widespread, and highly individ-

ease experienced by patients, rheumatoid arthritis and osteoarthritis patients face chronic diseases with no cure that mandate their adaptation to fluctuating levels of chronic pain and varied restrictions on their activities and mobility.

Although it is not possible to predict accurately the specific impact of arthritis on any individual patient, it is possible to identify problems that commonly occur. The use of a common patient problems model can guide the nurse in making a thorough assessment of the patient and organizing strategies for successful intervention.

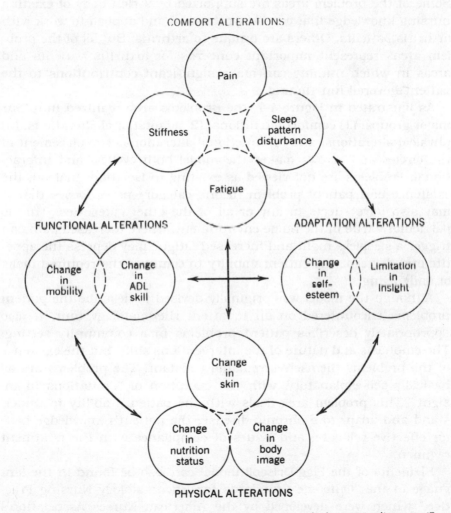

Figure 1–7. Frequently occurring problems in patients with rheumatic diseases. (From *Rheumatology Nursing*, Pigg, J. S., Driscoll, P. W., and Caniff, R. Copyright © 1985 John Wiley & Sons, Inc. Reprinted by permission of John Wiley & Sons, Inc.)

ualized. Despite significant differences in the degree of clinical dis-

Rheumatology nurses Pigg and Driscoll (1985) have developed a nursing model for conceptualizing the frequently occurring problems of patients with rheumatic diseases. The model deals with common patient problems and disease effects, rather than with medical diagnoses. An understanding of basic disease pathology as outlined in prior sections of this chapter is essential for care planning, but the nurse's role is focused on the effects of the disease rather than on the disease process itself. Nurses can make independent and important interventions in each of the problem areas identified in the model. Some of the problem areas are supported by a rich body of existing nursing knowledge that can be synthesized and applied to work with arthritis patients. Others are unique to arthritis. But all of the problem areas represent important concerns for arthritis patients and areas in which nursing can make significant contributions to the patient's overall functioning.

As illustrated in Figure 1-7, the problems are organized into four major groups: (1) comfort alterations, (2) adaptational alterations, (3) physical alterations, and (4) functional alterations. The placement of the circles and arrows makes the model both cyclical and interactional. Problems are not viewed as existing in isolation. Instead, the existence of a patient problem in one category presupposes that it may also have effects in any or all of the other categories. This is particularly true in the home environment, where increased pain can trigger a sleepless night and increased fatigue may depress the appetite and decrease the patient's ability to complete the required tasks of daily living.

Although the model was originally devised to describe the patient problems encountered on an inpatient rheumatology unit, it also appropriately describes patient problems in a community setting. The emphasis and nature of the interventions shift, but the existence of the problems themselves remains constant. The problems are all basically self-explanatory, with the exception of "limitations in insight." This problem area deals with the patient's ability to understand and adapt to a chronic disease; the patient's knowledge base for effective self-care; and issues of compliance with the treatment regimen.

Elements of the Pigg-Driscoll model can also be found in the language of the "Outcome Standards for Rheumatology Nursing Practice," which were developed by the American Nurses Association's Division on Medical Surgical Practice in 1983 and are reproduced in Table 1-4. The outcome criteria relate closely to the problem groups of

Table 1–4   American Nurses Association Outcome Standards for Rheumatology Nursing Practice, 1983

Standard 1

The individual incorporates pain management techniques into daily life.
Criteria: The individual:
1. verbalizes that pain is characteristic of rheumatic diseases.
2. identifies factors that exacerbate or influence pain response.
3. identifies changes in quality or intensity of pain.
4. establishes realistic pain relief goals.
5. verbalizes that pain often leads to the use of nontraditional and unproven self treatment methods.
6. identifies pain management strategies.
7. utilizes appropriate pain management measures.

Standard 2

The individual incorporates as part of daily activities those measures necessary to manage stiffness.
Criteria: The individual:
1. explains the relationship between stiffness and disease activity, medication, and activities of daily living.
2. verbalizes changes in the intensity and duration of stiffness.
3. describes appropriate methods for decreasing stiffness.
4. describes a schedule of daily activities which takes into account the intensity and duration of stiffness.
5. utilizes appropriate methods for decreasing stiffness.

Standard 3

The individual incorporates as part of daily activities those measures necessary to modify fatigue.
Criteria: The individual:
1. explains the relationship of fatigue to disease activity.
2. differentiates between psychological and physical factors that may cause fatigue.
3. identifies measures to prevent or modify fatigue.
4. utilizes measures to prevent or modify fatigue.

Standard 4

The individual achieves self-care independently or with the use of resources.
Criteria: The individual:
1. identifies factors that interfere with the ability to perform self-care activities.
2. identifies alternative methods for meeting self-care needs.
3. utilizes alternative methods for meeting self-care needs.

continued

Table 1–4 American Nurses Association Outcome Standards for Rheumatology Nursing Practice, 1983 (*Cont.*)

Standard 5

The individual attains and maintains optimal functional mobility.
Criteria: The individual:
1. identifies factors which interfere with mobility.
2. describes measures to prevent loss of motion.
3. utilizes measures to prevent loss of motion.
4. utilizes appropriate techniques and/or assistive equipment to aid mobility.
5. identifies environmental (home, school, work, community) barriers to optimal mobility.

Standard 6

The individual and family have necessary information about the disease process and the therapy to make self-care management decisions.
Criteria: The individual:
1. describes an appropriate plan for managing personal health care.
2. explains reasons for choices in personal management behaviors.
3. verbalizes sufficient information to meet self-management needs according to a personal value system.
4. identifies personal and community resources that may provide information or assistance.

Standard 7

The individual achieves a balance between the stress imposed by the rheumatic disease and personal fulfillment.
Criteria: The individual:
1. verbalizes psychological and physical stress factors.
2. identifies appropriate strategies for coping with personal stress.
3. revises expectations regarding amount and type of activity possible in daily life.
4. identifies available resources.
5. utilizes available resources.

Standard 8

The individual achieves a reconciliation between self-concept and the physical and psychological changes imposed by the rheumatic disease.
Criteria: The individual:
1. verbalizes an awareness that changes taking place in self-concept are a normal response to rheumatic disease.

Table 1–4   American Nurses Association Outcome Standards for Rheumatology Nursing Practice, 1983 (*Cont.*)

2. identifies strategies to cope with altered self-concept.
       The family:
1. verbalizes role changes.
2. identifies strategies to cope with role changes.

Copies of the Outcome Standards can be obtained through: American Nurses Association, 2420 Pershing Road, Kansas City, Missouri 63108.

Source: Reprinted with permission of American Nurses Association, 1983. *Outcome Standards for Rheumatology Nursing Practice*. Kansas City, MO: American Nurses Association.

the model and provide an excellent guide for both setting goals and measuring the effectiveness of interventions. These tools can be an excellent resource for care planning with arthritis patients.

An initial patient assessment tool developed from the language and concepts of the Pigg-Driscoll model is found in Table 1-5. Although additional detailed assessment material will be included in subsequent chapters, this tool provides a point of departure for the holistic assessment of the arthritis patient. It can be used as an interview guide to obtain the data necessary to begin to plan effective care. It will assist the nurse in identifying problems that are actively confronting the patient, eliminating those that are not a current priority.

The remainder of this book is organized into four parts corresponding to the four categories of problem groups of the Pigg-Driscoll model. Individual chapters address patient problems within those categories that are of particular importance to the care of the arthritis patient in the community setting. Not all of the identified problems will be discussed. The reader is referred to standard nursing references for appropriate interventions for patient problems with skin changes or changes in body image. Since the focus of this book is on home care, problems have been added to the functional alterations category to deal with sexuality concerns and to the physical alterations category to deal with rehabilitation concerns after total joint replacement.

Table 1–5   Initial Home Assessment for the Patient with Arthritis

   I. Patient's summary of the history and course of the disease process
  II. Medications in current use and schedule
 III. Patient's perceptions of priority problems at this time
  IV. Comfort alterations
    A. Pain
       1. Patient's subjective report of the pain experience: location, duration, severity
       2. Methods for home treatment
       3. Impact on work or leisure activities
       4. Objective presence of swelling, heat, guarded movement
    B. Stiffness
       1. Patient's subjective report of stiffness: location, duration, severity
       2. Methods for home treatment
       3. Impact on work or leisure activities
       4. Objective presence of restricted movement
    C. Fatigue
       1. Patient's subjective report of fatigue: duration, severity
       2. Methods for home treatment
       3. Impact on work or leisure activities
    D. Sleep pattern disturbance
       1. Patient's normal sleep pattern
       2. Changes caused by arthritis
       3. Methods for home treatment
       4. Impact on work or leisure activities
   V. Physical Alterations
    A. Change in nutritional status
       1. Weight and body build
       2. Patient's report of normal dietary pattern: meal size and schedule, food likes and dislikes, person responsible for shopping and cooking
       3. Assessment of patient's general nutritional status: skin turgor, muscle tone, mucous membranes, hair and nails
    B. Change in body image
       1. Patient's general appearance and grooming
       2. Presence of the complications and deformities of arthritis
       3. Patient's perceptions of physical self and of changes induced by arthritis
  VI. Functional alterations
    A. Change in mobility
       1. Patient's subjective assessment of mobility: capabilities and limitations, assistive devices in use
       2. Observations on posture, gait, and joint range of motion
       3. Current exercise regimen
       4. Impact of changes on work or leisure activities
       5. Impact of changes on sexual relationships

Table 1–5 Initial Home Assessment for the Patient with Arthritis (*Cont.*)

B. Changes in skills related to activities of daily living
  1. Patient's subjective assessment of degree of independence in bathing and oral hygiene, feeding, dressing, toileting
  2. Patient's perceived ability to manage home tasks: general housework, cooking, laundry, child care, driving, yard work, assistive devices in use
  3. Impact of changes on work and leisure activities
  4. Environmental assessment: home layout, stairs, presence of assistive modifications, safety precautions and hazards
  5. Degree of assistance from family members or friends available to patient
VII. Adaptational alterations
  A. Change in self-esteem
    1. Patient's family and social roles, assessment of relationships
    2. Impact of disease on ability to fulfill role requirements
    3. Patient's subjective assessment of personal coping style and strengths
    4. Knowledge of stress management techniques and ability to implement them in daily life
  B. Limitation in insight
    1. Patient's knowledge of the disease process and understanding of the treatment plan
    2. Patient's knowledge of and perceived compliance with medication regimen
    3. Patient's use of unproven remedies
VIII. Summary of patient's current status and initial problem list identification

CASE STUDIES

1. Clarence Ginder is 52 years old and has osteoarthritis in his right hip. He has a lot of pain, which worsens when he walks for any length of time. His other hip causes no problems. He is also extremely stiff and has trouble standing up straight. He begins to walk with a pronounced limp, but his gait improves slowly as he moves. He states that the pain and stiffness are irregular: "Some days they'll be real bad, and other days I'm pretty much okay." Aside from some occasional lower back pain, Mr. Ginder's other joints are in fairly good condition, and he continues to work full time.

  1. What features of Mr. Ginder's condition are typical of osteoarthritis? What features, if any, are not?
  2. Is his pattern of pain and stiffness typical or atypical?
  3. What other symptoms of osteoarthritis would you assess for?

2. Tracy Johnson was diagnosed with rheumatoid arthritis 2 years ago at the age of 23. The disease started with acute inflammation and pain in her left thumb, which persisted for weeks. She had no further symptoms of the disease until a few months ago, when she developed acute inflammation and pain in the MCP and PIP joints of the fingers on each hand. At its onset she also noticed general body aching and weakness, and she developed a low-grade fever that lasted for several weeks. Even now she doesn't have much energy and has to exert herself to meet her normal work and family responsibilities.

1. Does Tracy have a typical case of rheumatoid arthritis? Does it usually affect women of her age?

2. Was her initial symptom pattern typical? Did her initial condition meet the criteria for a diagnosis of rheumatoid arthritis?

3. Did Tracy's disease then follow a typical course? Why or why not?

4. What typical features does her disease exacerbation exhibit? Are there any unusual features?

PATIENT EDUCATION MATERIALS

Arthritis Foundation. (1983). *Rheumatoid arthritis*. Arthritis Foundation, 1314 Spring St., N.W., Atlanta, GA 30309.

Arthritis Society. (1984). *Facts about rheumatoid arthritis*. Arthritis Society, 920 Yonge St., Suite 420, Toronto, Ontario M4W 3J7, Canada.

Decker, J. L. (1982). *Arthritis*. National Institutes of Health, Clinical Center Office of Reports and Inquiries, Bldg. 10B, Room 5C305, Bethesda, MD 20205.

Engleman, E. P., & Silverman, M. (1979). *The arthritis book. A guide for patients and their families*. E. P. Dutton Publishers, 2 Park Ave., New York, NY 10016.

Fries, J. F. (1986). *Arthritis: A comprehensive guide to understanding your arthritis*. Addison-Wesley Publishing Company, Jacob Way, Reading, MA 01867.

Scott, J. T. (1981). *Arthritis and rheumatism: The facts*. Oxford University Press, 200 Madison Ave., New York, NY 10016.

AUDIO VISUAL MATERIAL

Arthritis Foundation. (1980). *Two different diseases: Osteoarthritis and rheumatoid arthritis*. Arthritis Foundation, 1314 Spring St., N.W., Atlanta, GA 30309.

Arthritis Society. (1982). *The disease is arthritis.* Arthritis Society, 920 Yonge St., Suite 420, Toronto, Ontario M4W 3J7, Canada.

Brigham and Women's Hospital. (1981). *Arthritis: Basic information.* Arthritis Foundation—Massachusetts Chapter, 59 Temple Place, Boston, MA 02115.

A complete, up-to-date annotated bibliography on arthritis may be obtained from the National Arthritis and Musculoskeletal and Skin Disease Information Clearing House, Box 9782, Arlington, VA 22209.

BIBLIOGRAPHY

American Nurses Association (1983). *Outcome standards for rheumatology nursing practice.* Kansas City, Mo.: American Nurses Association.

Dickenson, G. R. (1980). A home care program for patients with rheumatoid arthritis. *Nursing Clinics of North America, 15*(2), 403–418.

Ehrlich, G. E. (1980). *Rehabilitation and management.* Boston: Butterworth.

Fries, J. F. (1986). *Arthritis: A comprehensive guide to understanding your arthritis.* Reading, Mass.: Addison-Wesley.

Katz, W. A. (1986). *Rheumatic disease: Diagnosis and management,* 2nd ed. Philadelphia: J. B. Lippincott.

Kelly, N., Harris, E. D., Ruddy S., & Sledge, C. B. (eds.) (1981). *Textbook of rheumatology.* Philadelphia: W.B. Saunders.

Koerner, M. E., & Dickenson, G. R. (1983). Adult arthritis: A look at some of its forms. *American Journal of Nursing, 83*(2), 253–261.

Kushner, I., Forer, A., & McGuire, A. B. (eds.) (1984). *Understanding arthritis.* New York: Scribner's.

Lorig, K., & Fries, J. F. (1986). *The arthritis helpbook.* Reading, Mass.: Addison-Wesley.

Pigg, J. S., Driscoll, P. W., & Caniff, R. (1985). *Rheumatology nursing.* New York: Wiley.

Riggs, G. K., & Gall, E. P. (eds.) (1984). *Rheumatic diseases: Rehabilitation and management.* Boston: Butterworth.

Rodnan, G. P., Schumacher, H. R., & Zvaifler, N. J. (1983). *Primer on the rheumatic diseases,* 8th ed. Atlanta: Arthritis Foundation.

Scott, J. T. (1981). *Arthritis and rheumatism: The facts.* New York: Oxford University Press.

Appendix A

Referrals

Referrals are an important tool of community nursing practice. The services of various members of the interdisciplinary health care team may be needed at different times in the course of arthritis therapy and for different patient situations. Making a referral for additional services appears to be a straightforward intervention, but this is seldom the case. The referral process is particularly difficult when the referral is made to the mental health system.

The community health nurse needs to be aware of the resources that are available in the local community for dealing with the varied problems related to arthritis. Compiling a list of phone numbers and addresses is a useful initial step, but information on the financial, transportation, and scheduling aspects of each provider is also needed. Identifying specific individuals with interest or expertise in arthritis or chronic disease can be very helpful. Providing the patient with a specific person's name as well as the agency name increases the possibility of a productive referral. Other useful guidelines are the following:

1. Present the referral in a positive way: "I have talked with this person, and he has helped other people like you."

2. If possible, encourage a spouse, child, or friend to accompany the patient to the first appointment.

3. If you are concerned about the patient's ability to make the contact independently, make the call with or for the patient.

4. If you are concerned about self-destructive behavior, make the call for the patient immediately.

5. Obtain the patient's permission (a) to contact the referral source and educate this person about the patient's needs and (b) to follow up on progress.

6. Do not make the referral if you would be unwilling to use this service yourself. Be aware of the good providers in your community.

Appendix B

Contracting

A formal agreement or contract is sometimes useful in establishing self-help skills or encouraging compliance with a treatment regimen. The force of habit is strong. A formal commitment between two persons increases the probability that the goal will be met.

Contracts may be either informal or formal. When informal agreements fail, formal agreements are necessary. A formal contract has the following characteristics:

It is written.

The goal is defined.

The specific behavior to be performed is described in detail (what, how often, where, when).

The rewards for performing the behavior are spelled out in detail.

Before a contract is drafted, it is necessary to gather certain information. Does the patient genuinely wish to change, learn, or practice the skill in question? A contract should never be forced on a patient. A contract can only help someone achieve a goal. It cannot change a negative attitude. Does the nurse have time for follow-up? A contract needs to be monitored. While formal agreements are excellent tools for communication and motivation, they also require considerable effort by both parties. Only one goal or behavior should be contracted for at a time. Both parties should have written copies as reminders.

SAMPLE CONTRACT

I want to _____
                                                      (list goal)
To reach this goal, I will:

_____

_____

_____

_____ times per day/week for _____ days/weeks. At that time I will look at my progress. I make an agreement with _____ to uphold this promise.
                                        (Home Health Nurse's Name)

As a reward for helping myself, I will _____

_____ .

_____   _____
          (Date)   Patient's Signature
I commit myself to help _____ with this goal and will check with him/her _____ daily/weekly/monthly as a reminder that his/her health is important to me.

_____   _____
          (Date)   Community Health Nurse's Signature

2

Drug Therapy in Arthritis

Ann S. Goodson
Judith K. Sands

Drug therapy is one of the essential components of a comprehensive treatment plan for rheumatoid arthritis and osteoarthritis. A variety of drugs are available for use with arthritis patients, each acting in a slightly different way. They range from common over-the-counter substances such as aspirin to complex compounds such as immunosuppressive agents that attempt to induce remission in rheumatoid arthritis. Drugs are prescribed primarily to control symptoms such as pain and inflammation, but they are also administered in an attempt to halt the disease process. There is no sure way to predict how well a particular patient will respond to a specific medication, as individual responsiveness varies substantially. The specific drug action, dosage, administration schedule, and disease state all interplay in subtle ways. Optimal drug prescription requires time and patience of both the physician and the patient. The choice of which drugs to utilize will be based on the physician's best judgment about the nature of the disease process, the severity of the symptoms, and general factors such as the patient's age and overall health status.

It is essential that arthritis patients be knowledgeable about their medication regimen so that they can make informed decisions about compliance and self-care. A certain amount of trial and error is an inevitable part of the development of a successful treatment protocol. However, this process can be highly disconcerting to patients and can even shake their faith in the entire treatment approach. The nurse must assume an important role in the overall education of patients. An enormous amount of information is presented to newly diagnosed patients about their disease process, exercise prescriptions, medications, and other factors. When disease activity and anxiety are high, patients may comprehend and internalize only small amounts of this information. The nurse, particularly one who practices in the community, is in an excellent position to increase the patient's knowledge base steadily.

Noncompliance and limitations in insight are common medication-related problems that the nurse must deal with in the home environment. When patients are hospitalized, they are in a relatively controlled environment in which medications are taken specifically as prescribed by the physician. However, such control is not realistic in the home environment. Disease exacerbations and symptom flare-ups may cause patients to question the effectiveness of the drug regimen. Chronic side effects and prohibitive costs can be a strong deterrent to consistent drug administration. In addition, in the home environment, patients are bombarded with suggestions from friends and relatives, as well as with heavy media advertising that promises arthritis relief from the use of various remedies.

The arthritis treatment industry is a highly profitable one that invests millions of dollars in advertising, particularly through television. Well-known entertainers and impressive graphics team up to convince patients that there is "scientific evidence" that arthritis relief is waiting on the shelves of the local drug or grocery store. The over-the-counter market is an immensely profitable portion of the pharmaceutical industry, and each product is marketed to compete aggressively for its share of the profits.

The community health nurse must be prepared to assist patients and their families to be knowledgeable consumers. They must understand what is known about the treatment of arthritis and supported by research, and must be able to evaluate the claims of drug advertisements intelligently. Therefore the community health nurse must possess extensive knowledge about drug therapy in arthritis and must be able to use that knowledge to foster the patient's adherence to the prescribed drug regimen. The remainder of this chapter is devoted to a discussion of the various drugs used in arthritis treatment, their side effects, and the associated nursing implications for patient teaching.

PYRAMID APPROACH TO DRUG TREATMENT

Arthritis drug treatment uses both disease-specific and nonspecific medications. Figure 2-1 illustrates a commonly used approach to drug therapy in arthritis. The base of the pyramid is formed by rapid acting nonsteroidal anti-inflammatory drugs, which are extensively used in the treatment of both rheumatoid arthritis and osteoarthritis. They are not directed at the etiology of the rheumatic disease process, but they act very effectively against joint inflammation and its associated pain. The second-line drugs attempt to interrupt or modify the actual disease process and are generally used in the treatment of rheumatoid arthritis. Corticosteroids provide the most effective anti-inflammatory treatment available, but their use in arthritis treatment should be temporary through intra-articular injection or short-term systemic administration. Although they provide excellent symptomatic relief, corticosteroids do not halt the underlying disease process, and their serious side effects prevent their ongoing use in basic arthritis management. None of the drugs on the pyramid can

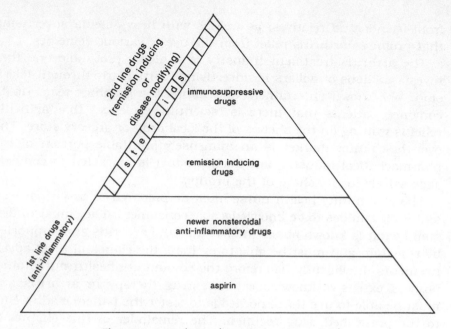

Figure 2–1. Arthritis drug treatment pyramid.

effect a cure, but they can make a significant contribution to interrupting the inflammatory process and relieving the symptoms of pain and stiffness.

Nonsteroidal Anti-Inflammatory Drugs

The nonsteroidal anti-inflammatory drug (NSAID) category includes both the salicylates and the rapidly growing group of newer NSAIDs that are used in arthritis therapy for both their anti-inflammatory and their analgesic actions. They are most commonly used as an ongoing part of therapy for chronic arthritis, but they may also be used on a more limited intermittent basis to manage or treat fluctuating periodic episodes of pain.

The NSAIDs can be classified according to their chemical composition, as shown in Table 2-1, but such classifications do not provide much insight into the specific clinical effects of the drugs. Within each drug category are potentially wide variations in specific effects, drug half-life, patient tolerance, and other factors. All NSAIDs inhibit the enzyme cyclooxygenase, and this action is believed to account for much of their antipyretic and analgesic effects. This inhibition of enzyme action also plays a role in their general anti-inflammatory

Table 2–1   Chemical Classification of Common NSAIDs

Salicylates
  Aspirin
  Other salicylates
Propionic acid derivatives
  Ibuprofen (Motrin, Bufren)
  Naproxen (Naprosyn)
  Fenoprofen calcium (Nalfon, Fenopron)
Indoles (indomethacin related)
  Indomethacin (Indocin, Indocid)
  Tolmetin (Tolectin)
  Sulindac (Clinoril)
Pyrazoles
  Phenylbutazone (Butazolidin)
  Oxyphenbutazone (Tandearil, Oxalid)
Oxicams
  Piroxicam (Feldene)
Fenamates
  Mefenamic Acid (Ponstel)
  Meclofenamate sodium (Meclomen)

effect but does not describe it fully. These drugs decrease vascular permeability and edema, and are believed to interfere with several stages of the inflammatory process, but these actions have not yet been clearly identified.

All of the currently available NSAIDs are effective for use in both rheumatoid arthritis and osteoarthritis, but their use varies. While they are prescribed on an ongoing basis in rheumatoid arthritis, their use in osteoarthritis may be continuous or intermittent on an as-needed basis, depending on the patient's symptoms. They are used primarily for their analgesic effects. Not all drugs, however, are effective in a particular patient. Individual responsiveness to specific drugs varies significantly, and there is no way to predict the effectiveness of any drug in advance from an individual patient's symptoms or disease course. Trial periods are usually required to determine which particular drug produces the optimal effect for any specific patient. This process may require several months and is inevitably frustrating, discouraging, and expensive for the patient. If all other factors are equal, variables such as cost and dosage schedule convenience will also be considered in the prescription decision. There is no evidence that combination therapy using two or more NSAIDs offers greater therapeutic benefit than one such drug used alone. NSAIDs can, however, be safely used with other analgesics and in combination with gold or penicillamine during the early stages of therapy.

Acetylsalicylic Acid (Aspirin)

Aspirin is usually among the first drugs prescribed for arthritis and may remain a mainstay of the treatment protocol for a long time. Aspirin was introduced clinically almost a century ago and over time has proven to be consistently effective as an analgesic and anti-inflammatory medication. Aspirin appears to produce its anti-inflammatory effects by interfering with the body's production of prostaglandins. It is an inexpensive drug, and therapeutic blood levels are relatively easy to obtain with adequate doses. The major drawback to aspirin therapy is the fact that 3.6 g daily is often required to establish therapeutic levels, and this amount is often associated with the development of significant side effects. Despite the incidence of side effects, however, aspirin continues to play a basic role in the management of arthritis.

Patients, however, may be less than enthusiastic about the idea of making aspirin the foundation of their medication treatment plan. They may have invested a great deal of time and money in a complete disease workup by a rheumatologist, and then to be instructed simply to take 10–16 aspirin daily may seem extremely anticlimactic. This lack of understanding about the use of one of the cheapest yet most effective arthritis medications can quickly lead to poor compliance with the drug regimen. The joint inflammation of rheumatoid arthritis responds slowly to aspirin. For this reason, the patient must achieve and maintain therapeutic drug levels on a daily basis. There is some correlation between plasma salicylate levels and drug effects, so a goal of treatment is to establish and maintain a plasma level between 20 and 30 mg/100 ml. This usually necessitates an adult dose of 900 mg (15 grains) four times a day. Patients must consistently take the full proper daily dose to maintain this therapeutic level in the blood. Patients who do not understand the drug regimen or do not believe in the effectiveness of aspirin and therefore repeatedly miss or skip doses are not likely to benefit from the use of salicylates. Patients with osteoarthritis use aspirin primarily for its analgesic effects and do not need to be concerned with maintaining plasma levels. All patients may become more committed to an aspirin regimen if they understand that 600 mg of aspirin taken orally provides approximately the same analgesic effects as 2 mg of morphine sulfate administered by injection.

Aspirin's interference with the production of prostaglandins is also responsible for some of its undesirable side effects. Gastrointestinal irritation is one of the most common side effects of high dose aspirin therapy. High concentrations of aspirin appear to strip the stomach mucosa of some of its protective mucus and produce local irritation. This effect is significantly enhanced when the aspirin tablets lodge directly against the stomach mucosa. Patients complain of indigestion, epigastric pain, and nausea, although actual peptic ulceration is fairly rare. In most cases, gastric irritation can be reduced fairly easily by encouraging the patient to take the drug with food, milk, an antacid, or at least a full glass of water. Numerous preparations have been developed and marketed to attempt to lessen or eliminate the gastric irritation of aspirin. Buffered and coated products are available, as well as liquids and derivative compounds such as choline salicylate (Arthropan) and combinations of choline and magnesium salicylate (Trilisate). Such products are usually fairly effective in dealing with gastric irritation but tend to negate one of aspirin's most significant advantages: its low cost. If at all possible, patients should be encouraged to attempt to prevent gastric side effects through food and liquid buffering.

There are also numerous aspirin substitutes on the market, and patients should be taught to read labels carefully. Products such as Tylenol, Datril, and Anacin-3 are all forms of acetaminophen that cannot be used in place of aspirin with rheumatoid arthritis because they do not possess aspirin's anti-inflammatory effects. Acetaminophen can be used with osteoarthritis, however, and to supplement basic pain relief as needed. Careful reading of labels also applies to dosage strength. Many products come in both regular (300 mg) and extra (500 mg) strengths. One form of coated aspirin (Easprin) comes in a 975-mg dose, but this preparation requires a physician's prescription. Patients should also be cautioned about using over-the-counter ibuprofen compounds such as Advil, Nuprin, or Medipren in place of aspirin. The decision to use one of these products for any purpose besides supplementary and occasional analgesia should be made by the physician. Table 2-2 lists some of the commonly available aspirin and acetaminophen products.

Aspirin inhibits the production of prothrombin and decreases platelet aggregation or stickiness, resulting in an increased potential for bleeding. For the otherwise healthy individual this usually causes

Table 2–2 Over-the-Counter Salicylate and Acetaminophen Products

Aspirin Products[a]	Features
Plain aspirin (acetylsalicylic acid)	Least expensive form—less than $1 per 100 tablets
Bayer	Microcoated for swallowing
Empirin	Coated aspirin
Bufferin	Aspirin plus two buffers
Ecotrin	Aspirin plus an enteric coating
Arthritis Pain Formula	Microcoated aspirin plus two buffers
Ascriptin	Aspirin plus two buffers
Excedrin	Combines aspirin, acetaminophen & caffeine
Vanquish	Combines aspirin, acetaminophen, caffeine, and two buffers

Acetaminophen Products[b]	Features
Tylenol	No significant differences among these products
Datril	
Panadol	
Anacin-3	
Percogesic	Acetaminophen plus phenyltoloxamine

[a]Aspirin may also be obtained in children's doses, liquid, chewable tablet, gum, and suppository forms.

[b]Acetaminophen may also be obtained in children's doses, liquid, chewable tablet, and suppository forms.

no problem, but it is a potentially serious side effect for anyone with a coagulation disorder. Aspirin should not be used by any patient who is receiving anticoagulant therapy. Gastric bleeding is the usual form of bleeding, and although frank hemorrhage is not common, patients may develop anemia from chronic minor blood loss. All patients need to be taught to report immediately the occurrence of spontaneous nosebleeds and bleeding gums, an increased incidence of bruising, blood in the urine, or tarry stools. They should be instructed to carefully read the ingredients labels of all over-the-counter preparations such as cold remedies, since many of them contain aspirin, which would add to the total daily dosage.

Tinnitus (ringing in the ears) and hearing loss are also possible side effects of high-dose aspirin therapy. The development of hearing problems has been shown to be dose related, but the threshold may vary substantially from patient to patient. Patients need to be alerted to the possibility of these side effects and instructed to reduce the total daily dose of aspirin if they occur. A 20% reduction, for example, from 15 to 12 tablets, is usually sufficient to control the symptoms.

In a minority of patients, aspirin therapy may aggravate asthmatic conditions or allergic rhinitis. Mild fluid retention may occur, which could interfere with the effectiveness of antihypertensive medication. A few patients experience a true allergy to aspirin, which can produce an anaphylactic reaction in susceptible individuals. Chemical derivatives such as diflunisal (Dolobid), choline magnesium trisalicylate (Trilisate), and salsalate (Disalcid) may occasionally be substituted successfully.

Aspirin toxicity is a serious potential complication of therapy, and patients must be aware of the warning signs. Serum salicylate levels above 30 mg/100 ml put patients at risk. Early signs include headache, sweating, dizziness, and tinnitus. Severe toxicity produces

---

Table 2–3 Teaching Interventions for the Patient on High-Dose Aspirin Therapy

1. Take the total prescribed dose of aspirin every day. Do not skip doses or days. It is essential to maintain therapeutic blood levels.
2. Take the aspirin in divided doses throughout the day every 4–6 hours. If a dose is missed, take it as soon as possible and reschedule the remaining doses.
3. Take the aspirin with a full glass of water. If stomach irritation develops, take the aspirin with food, milk, or antacids.
4. If stomach upset persists, try taking the dose at the end of a meal or using buffered or enteric-coated aspirin.
5. If hearing loss or ringing in the ears develops, do not stop taking the aspirin. Instead take 2–3 fewer tablets per day than your usual dose. The problem should stop within a few days. Slowly resume your prescribed dose. Contact your physician if hearing problems persist or if you have any questions about the dose.
6. Watch for and report any nosebleeds, bleeding gums, easy bruising, blood in the urine, or dark stools.
7. Read over-the-counter medicine labels carefully. Many of them contain aspirin. Many drugs also come in different strengths.
8. Do not substitute acetaminophen products (Datril, Tylenol) or ibuprofen products (Advil, Nuprin) for your aspirin. They can be used for occasional headaches or other temporary pain relief.
9. You can get aspirin in easy-open containers from your pharmacist. Ask for it.

nausea, vomiting, tremors, skin rashes, psychosis, and metabolic acidosis with hyperventilation. Immediate medical care is essential. Warning signs of aspirin toxicity should be provided to the family in writing and reviewed at regular intervals. Table 2-3 summarizes the teaching interventions appropriate for the patient receiving high-dose aspirin therapy.

Newer Nonsteroidal Anti-Inflammatory Drugs

The newer NSAIDs were developed in the attempt to find drugs that provide potent anti-inflammatory and analgesic effects and yet are not as irritating to the gastrointestinal tract. Many of the effects of these NSAIDs are similar to those of aspirin, but in some cases, fewer doses are required to reach and maintain therapeutic levels. This decreases the incidence and severity of the associated side effects and makes these drugs more convenient for patients to use. NSAIDs may be tried sequentially until a drug is found that provides the patient with the optimal effect. Patients need to understand that 2–3 weeks are required for each drug to begin to exert its full anti-inflammatory effect, so the process of exploration may well consume several months. Even when the newer NSAIDs are not successful in achieving an adequate disease response, they usually remain part of a patient's total drug protocol for anti-inflammation and analgesia.

Ibuprofen is the most widely known NSAID. It can now be purchased over the counter in nonprescription strength under a variety of trade names (Motrin, Bufren, Advil, Nuprin). Because the cost per tablet for the over-the-counter forms is lower than that of the prescription forms, patients may be tempted to substitute one of these products for their prescription drug. They must be cautioned to make cost comparisons by required dosage and not by the per tablet price. In its over-the-counter form, ibuprofen is sold in 200-mg tablets, whereas prescription ibuprofen comes in 400-, 600-, and 800-mg strengths. The increased number of pills required to achieve the prescribed dose may in fact cause the over-the-counter form to cost more, not less. Naproxen (Naprosyn) and fenoprofen (Nalfon) are other commonly prescribed NSAIDs with chemical compositions, side effects, and effectiveness quite similar to those of ibuprofen.

The most commonly reported side effects of these drugs are gastrointestinal: nausea, vomiting, heartburn, or diarrhea. These side effects can usually be fairly easily managed by taking the medications with food, milk, or antacids. Fluid retention due to prostaglandin blockage can also be a problem. Ibuprofen inhibits platelet aggregation but does not affect the prothrombin or whole blood clotting time. Oral anticoagulants can usually be used safely if the patient's status is carefully monitored. Patients should receive regular follow up care to monitor for any evidence of drug toxicity.

Indomethacin (Indocin), tolmetin (Tolectin), and sulindac (Clinoril) are another group of similar NSAIDs. They are all strong prostaglandin inhibitors and tend to produce a wider range of side effects than does ibuprofen. Indomethacin was widely used in the past but is less commonly employed today because of its frequent side effects. In addition to being monitored for gastrointestinal side effects, patients taking these drugs should be closely checked for signs of bleeding and the development of renal toxicity. These drugs have been shown to be ulcerogenic. Concurrent use of aspirin products should be avoided, as it increases the risk of bleeding and appears to decrease therapeutic blood levels.

Another group of NSAIDs includes mefenamic acid (Ponstel) and meclofenamate sodium (Meclomen). They tend to cause diarrhea, in addition to the standard gastrointestinal effects.

Piroxicam (Feldene) may be prescribed when ease of administration is a priority. It has a long half-life and deteriorates very slowly in the body. Therefore it can be administered on a once a day schedule.

The use of NSAIDs with elderly patients must be carefully monitored. Most of these drugs are excreted by the kidney and should be used cautiously in individuals with compromised renal function. The

Table 2–4 Teaching Interventions for the Patient Receiving Newer NSAID Therapy

1. Take the medication with food or an antacid. These drugs can be very irritating to the stomach.
2. If diarrhea occurs, keep your fluid intake high. Avoid gas-forming and high-fiber foods. If diarrhea persists, contact your physician.
3. Avoid the use of alcohol, which is also very irritating to the gastrointestinal tract.
4. Report any signs of blood in the urine or dark stools immediately.
5. Do not also take aspirin unless specifically instructed to do so by your physician. Read the labels of all over-the-counter medicines carefully.
6. If unexplained skin rashes appear, report them immediately to your physician.
7. If swelling occurs, try to limit your total daily intake of salt. Do not cut back on fluids.
8. Call your physician to report any rapid weight gain in excess of 2 pounds.
9. See your physician regularly for necessary blood tests to monitor for drug toxicity.

same is true in prescribing for patients with borderline liver function. The drugs with prolonged half-lives that are convenient for elderly patients are also the ones most likely to cause problems. If they are prescribed, they should usually be given in reduced doses. Table 2-4 summarizes the teaching interventions for patients receiving newer NSAIDs.

Remission-Inducing or Disease-Modifying Drugs

The next level of drug therapy involves the use of slow-acting, remission-inducing drugs. Their use is considered when the NSAIDs are unsuccessful in controlling the disease process. These drugs work very slowly and require several months before their effectiveness can be evaluated. They produce a gradual decrease in the overt symptoms of rheumatoid arthritis and help to control its systemic effects. In some cases, disease progression appears to be slowed or halted on x-ray films, although the complete mechanism of action of these drugs is not known. Patients continue to receive first-line therapy with NSAIDs while the use of disease-modifying drugs is initiated.

Gold Therapy
Gold therapy or chrysotherapy has been used to treat rheumatoid arthritis for over 50 years. Its mechanism of action is still not completely understood, but it appears to suppress the immune response and inhibit the release of lysosomal enzymes in the involved joints. Gold therapy is usually initiated when a patient experiences progressive disease involvement that is not responsive to first-line NSAIDs or shows evidence of developing deformity. Aurothioglucose (Solganal) and aurothiomalate (Myochrysine) are gold preparations that are administered intramuscularly and are associated with the development of significant side effects. Recently, a new gold preparation that can be administered orally, auranofin (Ridaura), has been released for general use.

The protocols for administering either intramuscular or oral gold preparations are strict because the side effects are potentially severe. Side effects appear to develop more slowly and less frequently with the oral preparation. The intramuscular protocol begins with a test dose of approximately 10 mg, followed in a week by 25 mg and then by subsequent weekly injections of 50 mg to a projected total of 1,000 mg. This schedule requires about 20 weeks. In many patients, a response is not noted until at least 750 mg has been administered.

Maintenance schedules are then tailored to the individual patient's response pattern but usually involve ongoing injections every 2–4 weeks. This is a demanding and time-consuming process, and patient compliance can be a problem. The advantages of an oral preparation in terms of patient acceptability are obvious.

The administration of intramuscular gold also demands very careful patient monitoring, especially during the first 20 weeks. The serious side effects most commonly encountered with gold therapy include renal toxicity and bone marrow suppression. Most patients are monitored with a weekly or biweekly hematocrit, white blood cell count, and platelet count, as well as urine protein tests before the administration of each dose.

The most common side effect of gold injection is the development of a skin rash, which may be severe and require a temporary halt in treatment. The typical skin reaction is a red macular or papular skin rash that first appears on the trunk and is quite itchy. Proteinuria is usually a fairly direct sign of glomerular inflammation caused by the gold and tends to appear more slowly than the skin rash. It may require termination of the treatment, although, if identified early, it can usually be reversed by decreasing the dose or temporarily discontinuing the treatment. Bone marrow suppression with resultant aplastic anemia or agranulocytosis is a rare but potentially fatal side effect in a few patients and necessitates immediate withdrawal of gold treatment.

Early experience with the oral gold preparation auranofin (Ridaura) has shown it to be quite effective in inducing remission in rheumatoid arthritis, although the effective blood levels are lower than those reached with the injectable form. Patients may be started on the oral preparation and then switched to the injectable form if an adequate response is not achieved. The usual dose is a 3-mg tablet twice each day. Auranofin is a safer drug and produces significantly fewer side effects. The most common side effect is diarrhea, which may be relatively mild and transient. The diarrhea can usually be successfully managed by diet modification. Patients are encouraged to include increased amounts of fiber and roughage in their diets to increase the bulk of the stool. Fluid intake should be increased to compensate for losses. A bulk-forming preparation such as psyllium hydrophilic muciloid (Metamucil, Hydrocil) may be used to regulate elimination. If the diarrhea is severe and unresponsive to these basic measures, the drug may need to be discontinued. Occasional skin rashes may also occur, but patients do not appear to experience seri-

Table 2–5   Teaching Intervention for Patients Receiving Gold Therapy

1. The full therapeutic effect of the drug may not be apparent for several months.
2. Be sure to keep your scheduled appointments for laboratory tests and therapy.
3. Report the development of a metallic taste in the mouth to your physician.
4. Report the development of easy bruising, nosebleeds, or blood in the urine or stool to your physician.
5. Maintain good oral hygiene and inspect your mouth daily for ulcerations.
6. Diarrhea may occur with oral gold therapy. Modify your diet to include increased amounts of roughage and bulk. You can also safely take a preparation such as Metamucil. If the diarrhea is severe or persistent, contact your physician.
7. If oral gold upsets your stomach, take it with food or an antacid.
8. Report the development of any itchy, red skin or rash to your physician. Rashes often appear on the trunk of the body.

ous bone marrow suppression. Auranofin causes gastrointestinal upset and should be taken with food. Some patients report a metallic taste in the mouth that may cause anorexia. Table 2-5 summarizes the teaching interventions appropriate for the patient receiving gold therapy.

Penicillamine

Penicillamine (Cuprimine, Depen) is a drug whose clinical effects are similar to those of gold salts. It has been shown to be effective in decreasing inflammation and stiffness in rheumatoid arthritis, as well as in slowing or interrupting disease progression. Its mechanism of action is basically unknown. It is slow-acting and requires at least 8–12 weeks to produce evidence of clinical improvement. Penicillamine produces multiple side effects and usually is employed when patients fail to respond to or cannot tolerate gold therapy.

Anorexia, nausea, and vomiting may occur early in the treatment program. Unlike other arthritis drugs, penicillamine should be administered on an empty stomach 30–60 minutes before a meal or 2 hours afterward. Patients usually require specific, repeated teaching on this aspect of therapy, since their other medications are routinely taken with meals. Gastrointestinal side effects are dealt with by keeping the daily dose low and allowing the patient to develop tolerance to it. Administering a full glass of water with the drug may help to resolve the problem. If anorexia or nausea persists, however, the penicillamine can be taken with food, although absorption will be less efficient. If the drug is taken with meals, patients should attempt to follow a consistent pattern each day in relation to their daily meal pattern.

Acute episodes of night fevers may occur in some patients after the first few doses of penicillamine. Since these fevers are a possible sign of an allergic response to the drug, they should be reported to the physician. The daily dose needs to be kept very low during this period.

Distortion or loss of the sense of taste is a relatively frequent drug side effect that can occur after about 6 weeks of therapy. Interference with the perception of salty or sweet tastes is particularly common. The problem usually resolves within another 6 weeks but can be very troublesome, particularly if patients also experience a metallic taste. It is especially important to ensure adequate nutrition during this period, and patients need reassurance that the problem is reversible. Penicillamine also interferes with the absorption of vitamin B_6, and supplemental pyridoxine throughout therapy is appropriate. For some patients, the supplemental pyridoxine is useful in decreasing or alleviating the taste problems.

Skin rashes with accompanying pruritis also frequently appear in the first months of therapy and are believed to be a sensitivity reaction. Drug therapy should be temporarily halted and then restarted at a lower dosage level. The pruritis can usually be treated safely and effectively with antihistamines. Skin rashes that appear after 6 months or more of penicillamine therapy are very difficult to treat and may require discontinuation of the drug. Although penicillamine is a derivative of the penicillin molecule, it can be successfully used with patients who are penicillin sensitive, but it must be initiated with great caution.

Proteinuria is a potentially serious side effect of penicillamine therapy that can appear after 4 months or more of treatment. It is due to the deposition of immune complexes in the glomeruli. It does not usually produce renal impairment in otherwise healthy kidneys and gradually lessens over time. All patients need to have their urine protein levels monitored regularly. Therapy is usually discontinued if these levels exceed 2 g in 24 hours. Penicillamine use is contraindicated in patients with underlying renal insufficiency.

Bone marrow suppression is another potentially serious side effect of penicillamine therapy. Thrombocytopenia can develop at any time during therapy, and, although usually fairly mild, it can become severe. Patients should be taught to report promptly any unexpected bleeding or easy bruising, particularly blood in the urine or stool. The platelet level usually responds promptly to a temporary discontinuation of the drug. Therapy can then be restarted at a lower level. General bone marrow suppression occurs infrequently but is very serious and requires that treatment be halted. Patients should be encouraged to report promptly the development of mouth ulcers, sore throats, or fevers that may reflect neutropenia. Blood counts are checked once or twice weekly during the first few weeks of therapy and then at least at monthly intervals.

Long-term use of penicillamine may occasionally produce a variety of autoimmune disorders. These include a neuromuscular weakness similar to myasthenia gravis, Goodpasture's syndrome, polymyositis, and drug-related lupus. The development of any of these syndromes requires discontinuation of therapy.

Penicillamine therapy is usually started with a daily dose of 250 mg, and the patient's response is carefully evaluated. After 1–2 months the dose is increased to 500 mg a day and the patient's response is reassessed. Doses as high as 1 g daily may occasionally be required to produce the desired effect. Once a positive response is achieved, the dose is gradually decreased to a maintenance level, which can be increased again in the event of disease exacerbation. Blood counts and urinalysis monitoring are continued throughout treatment. Table 2-6 summarizes the teaching interventions appropriate to the patient receiving penicillamine therapy.

Table 2–6   Teaching Interventions for the Patient Receiving Penicillamine

1. Take the drug on an empty stomach, if possible, with a full glass of water. Take it 30–60 minutes before or 2 hours after a meal.
2. If nausea develops and persists, take the drug at the same times each day with a small amount of food.
3. Report the development of any skin rash or itching to your physician.
4. Report the development of any bad or unusual tastes to your physician.
5. Supplement your diet with 10–20 mg vitamin B_6 (pyridoxine) daily.
6. Report any episodes of fever to your physician.
7. Maintain scrupulous oral hygiene, and inspect your mouth daily for ulcerations.
8. Report the development of easy bruising, nosebleeds, blood in the urine, or dark stools to your physician.
9. Continue to take your medication unless specifically instructed to stop by your physician. It is important that you come in as requested for blood and urine testing.

Hydroxychloroquine (Plaquenil)

Hydroxychloroquine (Plaquenil) was developed during World War II for the treatment of malaria. In 1957 it was demonstrated for the first time that the drug also suppresses synovitis and produces a functional improvement in patients with rheumatoid arthritis and systemic lupus erythematosus. It is hypothesized that hydroxychloroquine has an action similar to that of gold, but it is not able to halt the progression of the rheumatoid arthritis disease process, as seen on x-ray films. It may take 6 months before patients demonstrate a positive response to the drug.

Retinopathy can be a serious side effect of hydroxychloroquine use. Its development appears to be related to both the dosage and the duration of treatment. The first sign of retinal damage is usually a change in the patient's peripheral visual fields or a loss of red vision. These effects appear to be caused by deposition of the drug in the pigment layer of the retina. Professional eye examinations at 4- to 6-month intervals allow early detection of ocular lesions. The damage is usually completely reversible when caught at an early stage.

Hydroxychloroquine may also cause gastrointestinal upset and skin rashes, but it produces almost no liver and renal toxicities and does not require close monitoring of laboratory values. It is given in low doses of 200–400 mg daily for 6 months and is then reduced to a maintenance dose of 200 mg daily. The drug should be taken with meals. Table 2-7 summarizes the teaching interventions appropriate for the patient taking hydroxychloroquine.

Immunosuppressive Drugs

The fourth level of the drug therapy pyramid consists of the powerful and potentially hazardous immunosuppressive drugs. Disorders in

---

Table 2–7   Teaching Interventions for the Patient Receiving Hydroxychloroquine

1. Have your eyes examined by an ophthalmologist before starting the drug and then every 6 months thereafter or at intervals specified by your physician.
2. Call your physician immediately if you detect *any* change in your vision (blurring, halos around lights, fuzziness, or flashes).
3. Take the medication with food or an antacid to avoid gastrointestinal irritation.
4. Report the occurrence of skin rashes to the physician.
5. Use sunglasses outdoors if you become sensitive to bright light. The use of sunscreens may help to prevent the development of skin rashes.

immune system functioning clearly contribute to the destructive inflammatory processes of rheumatoid arthritis, and increased understanding of this pathophysiologic process has led to the growing use of immunosuppressive agents in the treatment of patients who do not respond to other therapies. Because of their serious side effects and potential for toxicity, the administration of immunosuppressives is usually restricted to patients with severe or potentially life-threatening disease. Although their beneficial effects are not completely understood, it is clear that immunosuppressive drugs can be of significant help to selected patients.

Immunosuppressive drugs were first developed for use as antineoplastic agents. Although there are several distinct groups of immunosuppressives, all of them act relatively nonspecifically as cell poisons, inhibiting various metabolic pathways and killing rapidly proliferating body cells. Because these drugs do not selectively inhibit just one aspect of the immune response, the entire body's defense system is ultimately compromised. Therefore patients are potentially vulnerable to a wide range of opportunistic infections and have an increased risk of developing malignancy. There are numerous drugs in the immunosuppressive category. The three that have been used most extensively in the treatment of rheumatoid arthritis include methotrexate (Folex, Mexate, MTX, Amethopterin) and cyclophosphamide (Cytoxan, Neosar, Procytox), which are primarily antineoplastics, and azathioprine (Imuran), which has its principal use in preventing transplant rejection.

Although they act quite differently, the immunosuppressive drugs share some common side effects and toxicities. They have the capacity to cause severe and even fatal reactions and demand careful monitoring. Bone marrow suppression is the most serious side effect of immunosuppressive drug use. Red cells, white cells, and platelets are all affected, which can produce serious anemia, neutropenia, and thrombocytopenia. The prevention of serious episodes of bleeding or infection is an ongoing concern. When patients receive daily therapy, the drug's effects are cumulative and blood counts must be monitored weekly. Patients must be carefully instructed to maintain scrupulous personal hygiene, including frequent oral care; avoid exposure to infection, when possible; observe for easy bruising or the development of petechiae; and promptly report any nosebleeds, gum bleeds, or evidence of blood in the urine or stool.

The immunosuppressive drugs also tend to be very upsetting to the gastrointestinal tract and may cause anorexia, nausea, abdominal pain, vomiting, or diarrhea. The drugs are usually administered with food to reduce distress, although the use of oral antiemetics may occasionally be indicated.

Immunosuppressive drugs have also been shown to have teratogenic potential and should not be used during pregnancy. Contraception and the importance of preventing pregnancy are important points to review with any female patient in the reproductive years.

Because of their potentially serious side effects, immunosuppressive drugs should be used only after patients have received appropriate teaching about their risks and benefits. Informed consent is essential. In addition to the general effects discussed, each of these drugs also possesses unique effects and toxicities that must be covered in the overall teaching plan.

Methotrexate

Although the use of methotrexate in rheumatoid arthritis is relatively new, it has been widely and successfully used in the treatment of psoriasis and psoriatic arthritis. This long-term experience has led to a fairly complete understanding of its effects. It has a low potential for malignancy and can be used with relative safety, since its effects are fairly predictable.

Methotrexate produces multiple side effects. It is irritating to the gastrointestinal tract and suppresses bone marrow function, which requires careful monitoring. Stomatitis occasionally develops. Alopecia occurs with higher doses, and patients may note thinning of their hair. The drug is metabolized by the liver and may trigger hepatitis, which can progress to cirrhosis. Liver function tests should be carefully monitored, and patients should be cautioned to limit strictly or eliminate their intake of alcohol.

Methotrexate may be given orally. A weekly dose of 5–30 mg may be prescribed, depending on the patient's response. It is given in three to four divided doses separated by intervals of at least 12 hours.

Azathioprine

Azathioprine (Imuran) has been widely and successfully used in the prevention and treatment of transplant rejection. It has recently been approved by the Food and Drug Administration (FDA) for general use in rheumatoid arthritis. Its clinical effectiveness is usually demonstrated after about 12 weeks, and patients are then maintained on the lowest possible dose that will sustain the remission of symptoms.

During the initial weeks of therapy, when azathioprine is administered in higher doses, patients are at substantial risk of developing infection from leukopenia. The drug does not, however, exert a significant depressant effect on platelet formation, and bleeding is not a serious concern. Patients must be extremely alert to the signs of opportunistic infections and maintain scrupulous personal hygiene routines. All patients should be monitored closely for the development of renal or liver toxicity, which are also problems at higher dose levels. Gastric irritation can usually be successfully managed by administering the drug with meals.

Azathioprine is administered orally. The usual daily dose ranges from 1.5 to 2.5 mg/kg, depending on the patient's response.

Cyclophosphamide

Cyclophosphamide (Cytoxan) is closely related to one of the earliest antineoplastic drugs—nitrogen mustard. It has been a part of cancer therapy for many years and is occasionally used in rheumatoid arthritis. It causes bone marrow suppression, which necessitates frequent blood count monitoring, as well as patient teaching to prevent or identify infections and bleeding.

One of the most common specific effects of cyclophosphamide therapy is inflammation of the bladder, which can result in bladder wall hemorrhage. The drug should be administered in the morning and a high fluid intake should be maintained throughout the day. If cyclophosphamide is taken at night, its metabolite remains in the bladder overnight, increasing the irritating effect. Routine urine testing is indicated to check for the presence of red blood cells.

Other effects of cyclophosphamide include hair loss, infertility, decreased sperm counts, and ovum damage. Patients need to receive specific contraceptive and reproductive counseling before and during therapy. Cyclophosphamide can be administered either orally or parenterally. The usual oral dose is 1.5–2.5 mg/kg/day. If given by intravenous bolus, the usual dose is 10–15 mg/kg at 3- to 4-week intervals. Table 2-8 summarizes the teaching interventions appropriate for patients receiving immunosuppressive drugs.

Corticosteroid Therapy

Corticosteroids are the last drug category included in the treatment pyramid. Steroids are placed to the side of the drawing to indicate that their use should be temporary. They should not be considered a routine part of drug therapy. They are primarily used locally through

Table 2–8   Teaching Interventions for Patients Receiving Immunosuppressive Drugs

1. The drug may cause loss of appetite, nausea, vomiting, or diarrhea. Report the development of any of these problems to your physician.
2. Take the drug with food or milk. Plan your meals for times of the day when symptoms are minimal. Try eating small meals more frequently. A light diet is often best. Avoid fried and fatty foods.
3. Ask your physician for an antinausea medication if stomach upset persists.
4. Avoid contact with persons who have colds or other infections. Report sore throats, fever, or any other sign of infection to your physician immediately.
5. Maintain scrupulous oral hygiene and inspect your mouth daily for ulcerations. Report the development of mouth ulcers to your physician. Use a soft toothbrush for oral hygiene. Avoid highly seasoned foods.
6. Report the development of easy bruising, nosebleeds, or blood in the urine or stool to your physician.
7. Be sure to utilize effective birth control measures during therapy. Pregnancy should be avoided.
8. Be sure to keep your scheduled appointments for laboratory tests.

Specific Teaching for Methotrexate

1. Avoid the use of alcohol during therapy, as it can increase the risk of liver damage.
2. Some hair loss may occur, but hair will grow back as the drug dose is lessened.

Specific Teaching for Cyclophosphamide

1. This drug is irritating to the bladder. Be sure to take it in the morning and drink at least 2 quarts of fluid during the day.
2. Report the development of pain or burning with urination or blood in the urine to your physician.
3. Hair loss may occur during therapy, but hair will regrow once the drug is discontinued. You may want to experiment with wigs, hats, and scarves.

intra-articular injection to treat acute inflammatory flare-ups in individual joints or for episodes of generalized disease activity that occur during the period of "buildup" for a remission-inducing drug.

The use of systemic corticosteroids [prednisone (Deltasone), methylprednisolone (Medrol)] remains a controversial and unresolved issue. Steroids clearly produce significant suppression of both humoral and cell-mediated immune responses, as well as potent anti-inflammatory effects. They can produce prompt, dramatic improvements in a patient's level of comfort and functional well-being. Most of the disease-modifying drugs discussed in prior sections require months of therapy to achieve a positive response. Corticosteroids can elicit improvement in a matter of days. But long-term steroid use is clearly associated with serious side effects that may not be fully reversible. Fluid retention, weight gain, hypertension, congestive heart failure, diabetes, and osteoporosis are all potential effects of long-term use. It is generally recommended that systemic steroids be used conservatively on a temporary basis only to deal with the disabling effects of disease exacerbations or to support patients until one of the slower-acting drugs can effectively control the inflammatory process. Patients typically are quite familiar with the use of systemic steroids for arthritis treatment but are not usually as familiar with their long-term negative consequences. They may therefore request the use of steroids quite early in the disease management process. The doses required to control the symptoms of arthritis almost always lead to the development of Cushing's syndrome and need to be highly individualized.

The direct injection of steroids into the joint has played an important role in arthritis management for many years. Hydrocortisone acetate (Caldecort, Cortifoam, Hydrocortone) and triamcinolone (Aristospan, Amcort, Triam Forte) are commonly used. These preparations allow minimal systemic absorption of the drug. Intra-articular injection is used as an adjuvant to overall therapy for relief of inflammation and pain when just one or a few joints are involved. It brings an extremely potent agent directly into a confined space, bypassing the hazards of systemic use. Although a palliative measure, it is obvious that intra-articular injection produces dramatic and sometimes long-term relief for some patients. Steroid injection should not be used with badly damaged or infected joints. The dosage used ranges fairly widely, based on the size of the joint and the degree of inflammation.

A general principle for the administration of intra-articular steroids is that the longer the interval between injections, the better. Concern exists that frequent administration can cause rapid joint breakdown. Eight to twelve weeks is the minimum interval recommended, with 4–6 months preferred between injections into major weight-bearing joints. Improvement may be so dramatic following injection that patients need to be cautioned not to overuse the joint. Limited activity is usually recommended for a few days, although patients are permitted to move around.

Extensive patient teaching should accompany the extended use of systemic steroids, since the side effects are numerous. Patients usually experience weight gain as a result of sodium and water retention, as well as increased appetite. The characteristic redistribution of body fat may produce a significant alteration in the patient's appearance. Facial roundness, a buildup of fatty tissue on the trunk, and the development of a cervicodorsal fat pad at the base of the neck are all typical changes. Patients should follow a low-sodium diet and may need instruction concerning diet modifications to restrict their total

Table 2–9 Teaching Interventions for Patients Receiving Corticosteroid Therapy

Systemic Use

1. The medication should be taken with meals or antacids to reduce gastric irritation.
2. Report any incidence of epigastric pain or burning or the presence of blood in the stool to your physician.
3. Modify your diet to counter common side effects of the drug. Eat a diet high in potassium and protein; ensure adequate calcium intake; and eat a diet low in total calories and sodium.
4. Monitor your weight daily and report any weekly weight gain of 4–5 pounds to your physician.
5. Have your blood pressure monitored regularly.
6. Return for blood sugar monitoring as instructed by your physician.
7. Be aware of the possibility of changes in your appearance, including rounded face, muscle wasting in the extremities, thickened trunk, thinning of skin, and easy bruising.
8. Maintain scrupulous personal hygiene. Be alert to the development of infections and treat all skin injuries aggressively. Report sore throats or fever to your physician promptly.
9. Be alert to the possibility that the medication may cause mood alterations such as depression or euphoria.
10. Never discontinue your use of steroids abruptly. These drugs must be gradually tapered.
11. Carry Medic Alert identification indicating that you take steroid medication.

Intra-articular Injection

1. Follow your physician's instructions about using the affected joint carefully. Overuse can cause joint damage.
2. Report the development of pain, swelling, and heat at the injection site to your physician immediately.

caloric intake. The diet should also be rich in potassium, as this electrolyte is excreted when sodium is conserved. Patients need to be monitored closely for the development of hypertension. The chronic fluid excess also increases the potential for congestive heart failure.

Long-term steroid use also produces osteoporosis and significantly increases the risk of pathologic fractures, especially in the vertebrae. Patients must be taught to move with care and avoid strenuous activities that may result in fractures. Muscle wasting also occurs in the extremities, and patients should be taught to make sure that their diet contains an adequate amount of protein. Steroids are strongly ulcerogenic and should be taken with food or an antacid. Patients need to be monitored closely for signs of bleeding. Some patients also develop glucose intolerance while on steroids and need to be monitored carefully for glycosuria and hyperglycemia.

It is also essential that patients be taught never to stop taking steroid medications abruptly. Steroid use must be gradually tapered to allow the body to reestablish its own diurnal pattern of secretion. The abrupt withdrawal of systemic steroids can trigger an adrenal crisis and vascular collapse. Patients also need psychologic support during the period of discontinuation of steroid medication. These drugs offer such fast and effective relief that it is often difficult for patients to believe that long-term use is highly detrimental. Patients must be offered significant encouragement and support during this difficult process. Table 2-9 summarizes the basic teaching interventions appropriate for patients receiving corticosteroid therapy.

NURSE'S ROLE IN DRUG THERAPY

Community health nurses are an important resource for patients and families attempting to understand and cope with the complexity and uncertainty of arthritis drug therapy. The drug treatment protocol can be complicated and multifaceted, especially for patients with rheumatoid arthritis. In addition, its inherent uncertainties make it even more challenging for patients. Weeks or months of time and a substantial amount of money may be invested in a drug that may ultimately prove to be ineffective. The process is not only potentially very discouraging but may cause patients to wonder whether the entire area of drug therapy should not be more appropriately placed under the heading of "unproven treatments."

Patient education is clearly the primary role for nurses in drug therapy. Arthritis centers and physicians attempt to provide comprehensive teaching about prescribed drugs, but this teaching typically must take place during one or two concentrated sessions. The bulk of the teaching is provided verbally, which fosters uncertainty about what has been understood or will be retained. When patients are at home, the responsibility for their medication regimen falls squarely on themselves and perhaps on their family. Information about medications is frequently forgotten. Research indicates that elderly patients, in particular, are not likely to understand the purpose of their drug therapy even if they are conscientiously attempting to follow the protocol (Smith & Andrews, 1983). Assuming responsibility for knowledgeable self-care becomes a reality when patients confront the need to interpret and manage the side effects of drugs. These side effects can appear to be both serious and frightening, especially with disease-modifying or immunosuppressive drug therapy.

Compliance with treatment and drug therapy regimens is a well-researched area of concern. Attention has focused particularly on chronic illnesses such as hypertension, coronary artery disease, diabetes, and arthritis, where lifestyle modifications and drug therapy are essential components of the regimen. Although the research results are mixed, they do provide some general guidelines for effective interventions.

Patients must have written as well as verbal instructions about their drugs. Drug information that is transferred to index cards can be conveniently stored in small recipe boxes, readily available for referral as needed. Nurses should review or clarify drug information as needed at each contact with the patient and communicate any drug-related concerns promptly to the referring physician. All patient teaching materials should include important warning signs of adverse drug reactions or toxicities, plus specific instructions about what to do if they occur. This is particularly important when a drug regimen has been prescribed by physicians in an arthritis center that is not located in the local community. Drug information should be as complete but as uncomplicated as possible and should be carefully prepared, taking into consideration the patient's intellectual and educational levels. The regimen should be analyzed for unnecessary complexity. If a patient is experiencing difficulty with adherence, the nurse may need to explore with the physician ways to modify the drugs or doses in order to reduce the complexity of the schedule. The community health nurse should also know about other resources that are available in the community, including a reputable pharmacist for consultation, drug education classes, and the local poison control center.

Community health nurses can also assist patients to prepare and maintain a medication history. It should include information about drugs that have been prescribed, such as the dates started and discontinued, the side effects experienced, and an assessment of the drugs' effectiveness. A complex arthritis situation is very likely to be managed by several physicians over time, especially in our transient society. A careful and complete drug history makes drug information accessible to all health care providers, including dentists, and frees patients from complete dependence on the medical history that may be maintained at an arthritis treatment center. Most large chain pharmacies also have the capability to establish and maintain computer drug histories for patients. Patients should be encouraged to establish such a history with a reputable pharmacist and should be consistent in having all prescriptions filled at this individual's pharmacy. This introduces another professional resource to the patient's drug regimen and provides additional backup if the community health nurse's involvement with the family is short term. An example of a medication history form is shown in Figure 2-2.

Community health nurses also need to work with patients and families to find methods that will foster compliance with the drug regimen. Elderly patients and those who live alone are at particular risk for adherence problems. The family can be an important and effective resource, but it is essential that the drug regimen not become the focus of a battle in the home. Each patient situation presents unique demands, but there are several well-established strategies that may be helpful. Requesting packaging of drugs in easy open rather than child-resistant containers can significantly improve compliance. If young children are present in the home, this strategy must be coupled with adequate precautions to keep drugs out of their reach.

The nurse should ask patients how they remember to take their drugs. Refrigerator checkoff sheets and calendars can facilitate this process. Suggestions to associate drug doses with meals, snacks, or other activities are usually helpful. There are commercial drug dispensing trays for assisting patients to prepare and take their medications properly, but the nurse can easily create pill trays out of egg boxes or ice cube trays. Keeping drug bottles in accessible places such as the kitchen rather than the bedroom or bathroom can also be an effective technique.

Figure 2–2 Sample Medication History

Drug Name	Dose and Schedule	Date Started	Date Ended	Side Effects Experienced	Effectiveness

The nurse should also ensure that the patient has adequate resources to maintain the prescribed regimen. This is particularly important for elderly patients on fixed incomes. Lack of money is a common impediment to drug compliance as patients attempt to skip doses and stretch the duration of prescriptions. The nurse should direct patients to pharmacies that offer the lowest prices, as well as discounts for senior citizen and other groups, and instruct them to always specify their desire for generic drugs. Finances are an ongoing problem, however, as many prescription arthritis medications have a high price tag.

The community health nurse may also play a direct role in administering and monitoring the drug regimen, especially in rural areas. Most of the disease-modifying and immunosuppressive drugs require ongoing blood and/or urine monitoring. Particularly when patients are located some distance from the referral arthritis center, the nurse may be responsible for initiating and documenting the monitoring process. She may be ordered to administer the prescribed gold injections. The nurse must have a solid understanding of the drugs in use and their expected or potential side effects. A detailed protocol should be provided by the supervising physician concerning the nature and frequency of tests to be run, as well as the conditions that indicate a need for referral or intervention. In these situations, the nurse acts as the primary resource for patients and families concerning the drug protocol.

Perhaps the most important role of the community health nurse is to provide ongoing support to patients and families. Patients naturally experience periods of intense discouragement with any chronic, progressive disease process, and research indicates that compliance with chronic disease regimens tends to worsen over time. Concerns need to be verbalized and explored. A carefully thought-out education plan can support patients in their efforts to take charge of their disease process and cope effectively. The Arthritis Foundation is an excellent resource for information concerning drug therapy. A sample of these resources is included after the case studies at the end of the chapter. By fostering an ongoing commitment to the prescribed drug regimen, nurses can assist patients to evaluate unproven remedies intelligently. They can also support patients as advocates with physicians when symptoms exacerbate or become uncontrolled. Drug therapy is a critical component of disease management, and community health nurses are essential to its successful implementation.

CASE STUDIES

1. Mrs. Mary Russo is a 34-year-old woman who has recently been diagnosed as having rheumatoid arthritis. The disease started in the joints of her hands. Her physician prescribed aspirin—12 tablets daily in divided doses. Mary takes her medication erratically. She has young children and says, "I have to keep it out of their hands, and then I just forget it completely. I always take it, though, on days when I wake up feeling real sore." The family has a very limited income, and the cost of managing Mary's disease is of serious concern to them. She is buying small bottles of Ascriptin, saying, "This is supposed to be the best, but it's so expensive that I can only buy a little at a time."

   1. What do you consider to be the major problems in Mrs. Russo's understanding of and compliance with her drug regimen?
   2. What kind of a teaching plan would you develop? What content should be covered?

3. What strategies might you discuss to help Mrs. Russo with the issue of compliance?

4. What can you suggest to help her control the cost of her treatment?

2. Mrs. Ellen Perry is a 62-year old woman who has had rheumatoid arthritis for almost 20 years. She had very few symptoms of the disease during the first 10 years, but over the last 5 years her condition has steadily worsened. The disease process was not successfully controlled with any of the NSAIDs. She had a period of good response to gold, but recently the disease has exacerbated. Her physician suggests a trial with azathioprine (Imuran), but she is afraid to agree to this therapy.

1. What factors should Mrs. Perry be assisted to consider in making her decision? What does she need to know about azathioprine?

2. What are the risks and benefits of azathioprine? What side effects would she need to be aware of?

3. If she decides against using the drug, what other options does she have? What are their advantages and disadvantages?

4. If she decides to proceed with azathioprine therapy, what steps can she take to minimize the associated risks?

PATIENT EDUCATION MATERIALS

Arthritis Foundation. (1982). *Gold treatment in rheumatoid arthritis.* Arthritis Foundation, 1314 Spring St., N.W., Atlanta, GA 30309.

Arthritis Foundation. (1982) *Medication Brief Series: questions and answers about azathioprine, corticosteroids, cyclophosphamide, hydroxychloroquine, ibuprofen, indomethacin, meclofenamate, methotrexate, naproxen, penicillamine, phenylbutazone, sulindac, and tolmetin.* Available from the Arthritis Foundation, 1314 Spring St., N.W., Atlanta, GA 30309.

Arthritis Foundation. (1983). *Aspirin and related medications.* Arthritis Foundation, Public Education Department, 1314 Spring St., N.W., Atlanta, GA 30309.

Frankel, E. (1982). *Drugs, from ampicillin to zyloprim.* Atlanta, Ga.: Lupus Horizons. Lupus Erythematosus Foundation, 2814 New Spring Rd., Room 304-A, Atlanta, GA 30339.

Lages, W. F. (1985). *Arthritis drug fact sheet.* Arthritis Foundation— Northern California Chapter, Building 3—Suite 363, 185 Gerry St., San Francisco, CA 94107.

McKenna, C. H. (1978). *Penicillamine.* Arthritis Foundation—Minnesota Chapter, 122 W. Franklin Ave., Suite 440, Minneapolis, MN 55404.

Sack, K. E. (1979–81). *Drug cards.* Rosalind Russell Arthritis Center, University of California—San Francisco, 1442 Fifth Ave., San Francisco, CA 94143.

BIBLIOGRAPHY

Bunch, T. W., & O'Duffy, J. D. (1980). Disease modifying drugs for progressive rheumatoid arthritis. *Mayo Clinic Proceedings, 55,* 161–179.

Daniels, L. (1980). How can you improve patient compliance? *Nursing 80, 80*(5), 40–47

Goldenberg, D. L., & Cohen, A. S. (1986). *Drugs in the rheumatic diseases.* Orlando, Fla.: Grune & Stratton.

Heuberger, G. B. (1984). The role of the nurse with arthritis patients on drug therapy. *Nursing Clinics of North America, 19*(4), 593–604.

Huskisson, C. E. (1979). Antirheumatic drugs. *Clinics of Rheumatic Diseases, 5,* 351–736.

Marwick, C. (1982). All those arthritis drugs: How do you choose? *Medical World News, 23*(16), 58, 63–64, 69–72, 80.

Rodnan, G. P., Schumacher, H. R., & Zvaifler, M. J. (1983). *Primer on the rheumatic diseases,* 8th ed. Atlanta: Arthritis Foundation.

Sack, K. E. (1981). *Drug cards.* San Francisco: Rosalind Russell Arthritis Center.

Simon, L. S., & Mills, J. A. (1980). Nonsteroidal antiinflammatory drugs. *New England Journal of Medicine, 30,* 1179–1185.

Smith, P., & Andrews, J. (1983). Drug compliance not so bad, knowledge not so good—the elderly after hospital discharge. *Age & Aging, 12,* 336–342.

Spencer, R. T., Nichols, L. W., Waterhouse, H. P., & West, F. M. (1986). *Clinical pharmacology and nursing management,* 2nd ed. Philadelphia: J. B. Lippincott.

Strand, C. V., & Clark, S. R. (1983). Drugs and remedies. *American Journal of Nursing, 83*(2), 266–269.

PART 2

FUNCTIONAL ALTERATIONS

FUNCTIONAL ALTERATIONS

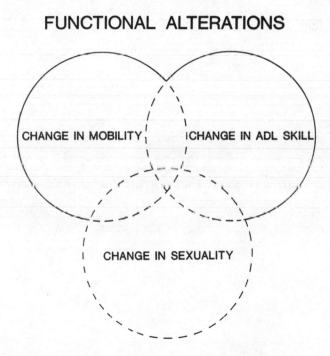

3

Changes in Mobility and Daily Living Skills

Cynthia Stabenow Kulp

Arthritis treatment programs clearly focus on improving or preserving patients' functional capacities. Therefore, the area of activities of daily living (ADL) receives heavy emphasis. This is particularly true for patients who are encountered or followed in the home setting, to whom community health nurses can make a significant contribution. Adults with mild or moderate disease may have barely acknowledged its impact on their daily living skills. Even patients with advanced disease may not have been assisted to perform a systematic assessment of the effects of their arthritis or introduced to methods of modifying the stress of the demands of daily living on their joints. The community health nurse has a wealth of specific, effective, and inexpensive strategies to employ with these patients.

ASSESSMENT OF ADL IN THE HOME

Successful nursing intervention in the area of ADL begins, as always, with a thorough and detailed assessment. This assessment provides the starting point from which an effective care plan can be developed. It also establishes a baseline for evaluating and measuring changes that may occur after intervention.

Since the community health nurse has the unique opportunity to work with patients in their homes, she is able to assess directly for ADL problems in this environment. This careful assessment provides the basis for appropriate problem solving and for the optimal positioning of equipment to facilitate patient activities.

Melvin (1982) outlines the opportunities that are afforded by an on-site home visit:

1. Assess the quality of home life in terms of family attitudes, interpersonal relationships, cooperation, and stress factors that significantly influence patient compliance with therapy.
2. Give the patient specific instructions on how to adapt the furniture or home to minimize joint stress and improve function.
3. Assess for architectural barriers in the home that may limit the patient's functional independence.
4. Assess the ease or difficulty of maintaining the house and yard.

The assessment procedure can take several forms: an interview, observation of the patient's activities, or a patient self-report. Usually a complete assessment involves a combination of all three. Regardless

Table 3–1 ADL Assessment

	Easily	With Difficulty	Not at All

BEDROOM: Can you . . .
1. Move from place to place in bed?
2. Roll to right/left side?
3. Turn and lie on abdomen?
4. Sit up in bed?
5. Get into/out of bed?

DRESSING: Are you able to put on and take off the following articles . . .

Women

    bra
    panties
    slip
    socks
    shoes
    blouse
    skirt
    sweater
    slacks

Men

    undershirt
    shorts
    trousers
    shirt
    sweater
    socks
    shoes

BATHROOM: Can you . . .
1. Get on and off toilet?
2. Adjust clothing?
3. Use toilet paper?
4. Flush toilet?
5. Maneuver bedpan?
6. Get to toilet at night?

BATHING: Can you manage . . .
1. Getting into/out of a bathtub/shower?

Table 3–1   ADL Assessment (*Cont.*)

	Easily	With Difficulty	Not at All
2. Turning taps on/off?			
3. Washing/drying all parts of body?			
PERSONAL CARE: Can you manage . . .			
1. Brushing teeth?			
2. Using a razor?			
3. Cutting: fingernails/toenails?			
4. Brushing and combing hair?			

Source: Reprinted with permission from ADL assessment—Canadian Arthritis and Rheumatism Society, in J. L. Melvin, *Rheumatic disease: Occaptional therapy and exercise*, 2nd ed. Philadelphia: F. A. Davis, 1982.

of the approach used, it is necessary to determine whether the patient is currently independent in terms of ADL or requires assistance to accomplish them. The assessment attempts to identify any stressful patient activities that could cause joint damage. It attempts to determine whether or not the patient is currently attempting to plan and pace daily activities to avoid undue fatigue and joint pain. Finally, it identifies any adaptive devices or methods that the patient is presently using to perform basic home activities.

When an occupational therapist is available to the home care agency, this professional can complete the detailed home assessment. In the absence of such interdisciplinary backup, however, the nurse can use or adapt a guide such as that shown in Table 3-1. This instrument can be used as an interview tool or can be left behind for the patient to complete and discuss with the nurse at the next home visit. The sample assessment presented here is limited to bed mobility, dressing, bathing, and personal care. A complete assessment would include cooking, routine housework, and home maintenance as well. Examples of complete, detailed assessments can be found in Melvin (1982), Pedretti (1985), and Trombly and Scott (1977).

Certain factors that are common to all rheumatic disease patients require special consideration in the ADL assessment. The first is morning stiffness. The nurse should determine its duration, location, and severity. Often patients say that they are able to dress themselves after lunch but are unable to do so first thing in the morning. The second factor is the percentage of "good" versus "bad" days. Patients who feel good one day may tend to overdo, and the result may be confinement to bed on subsequent days, unable to perform any activities. The nurse should also establish the time of onset and the duration of fatigue experienced by the patient with arthritis. Pain, anemia, and general deconditioning from inactivity can all contribute to a feeling of fatigue or lack of energy. The timing and dosage of medications both affect the patient's ability to tolerate an increase or decrease in activities at home. This is particularly true with corticosteroid medications.

Once the home environment has been assessed, the patient, nurse, physical therapist, and occupational therapist, can jointly plan an intervention program. The components of the program may vary significantly from patient to patient, depending on the severity of the disease process and the individual situation, but virtually all programs include the incorporation of joint protection principles, the use of assistive devices, and a home exercise program.

JOINT PROTECTION AND ENERGY CONSERVATION

The purpose of joint protection is to reduce stress and pain in the involved joints, and consequently to reduce inflammation and preserve the integrity of the joint structures. The incorporation of energy conservation training helps the patient conserve physical resources and improve functional endurance.

Although formal studies on the effectiveness of joint protection strategies have not been published, this can be readily demonstrated by specific patients who have learned to use two hands to perform an activity, or who invent an adaptive aid to meet their unique needs, or who learn to ask for help from family members. All of these strategies are part of the overall concept of joint protection.

Patient teaching about joint protection needs to be individualized to each patient's unique disease process, social situation, and physical environment. Although specific rules are usually not useful, as they apply to only a limited number of patients, there are general principles that have broad application. Silwa (1982) advocates the teaching of guidelines and general concepts, rather than specific dos and don'ts.

Regardless of whether a patient is newly diagnosed or has had rheumatoid arthritis for many years, the concepts of synovitis and cartilage destruction may not be completely understood. Yet these concepts provide an essential foundation for the application of joint protection principles. The nurse should attempt to explain the rationale for and value of joint protection based on the inflammatory process. The Arthritis Foundation is an excellent resource for a variety of reference materials that can assist in the education of patients with varied cognitive and educational levels. Some of these references are listed at the end of Chapter 1.

The nurse should teach the patient how to recognize and monitor the signs and symptoms of inflammation, namely, pain, warmth, and swelling. This may be the most important aspect of the patient's self-care program. Patients who can accurately and correctly identify periods of increased or decreased disease activity are able to appreciate the benefits of joint protection methods. They gain flexibility in monitoring and adjusting their medication program, increasing or decreasing their ADL tasks appropriately, and adjusting their exercise program in response to their disease status. They also gain positive reinforcement, which is invaluable in encouraging them to continue to use joint protection strategies.

Principles of Joint Protection

The basic principles of joint protection were first outlined for occupational therapists by Cordery (1965). These principles are still current, but they are only general guidelines. The individual strategies for implementing these principles are the responsibility of the professionals who work with rheumatic disease patients.

Balance Between Rest and Work

Whether the patient has a systemic or a degenerative disease, making choices among activities on a daily or weekly basis is the most difficult part of the total home care program. When patients have a chronic disease, they often do not realize the toll that chronic pain can exact while performing daily activities. Usually on a good day the patient tries to do everything at once, and happy family members often encourage the increased activity level. The nurse must emphasize the importance of daily, ongoing activity pacing, carefully balancing activities with rest periods. A day's or week's activities should be thoughtfully planned and scheduled. Simply reacting to the day's events will ultimately result in overfatigue and joint stress.

It is important for the patient to understand that it may be necessary to incorporate increased daytime rest periods into the home program. Patients who lose sleep at night due to joint pain or stiffness may need to catch up on their rest during the day. It is difficult to overemphasize the importance of appropriate rest. As Melvin has noted (1982), "The practice of resting before one becomes tired or exhausted is so effective that it should be the number one priority in energy conservation instruction. Once a person employs this practice the benefits are usually self-evident" (p. 354).

The long-term nature of the disease process requires that these behavioral changes become a part of the patient's daily routine almost for life. Behavioral change takes time and requires frequent reinforcement from both family members and professionals.

The most effective strategy to increase functional endurance is to rest before becoming exhausted. Taking a 5- to 10-minute rest during activities is difficult but can significantly increase overall functional endurance. The concept of resting for 10 minutes in the middle of an activity is totally foreign to the majority of adults. This practice lengthens the total time spent doing housework or yard work, and the desire to "get this over with" is usually strong. Yet sitting for only a few minutes before becoming tired will greatly increase one's total endurance. In addition, rest breaks during work provide more energy later on for the activities the patient enjoys.

The patient may need assistance with setting priorities for a day's or a week's activities. Before the onset of arthritis, the patient may have been physically active, involved in multiple community and leisure activities. Now the pace of such a schedule leaves the patient exhausted and hurting. Early in the home care program, it may be necessary for the nurse to assist the patient to plan and set priorities for the week. A return visit lets the patient and nurse examine the weekly calendar, monitor the signs of disease activity and joint pain, and modify the program as needed. A consistent balance is difficult to achieve, and patients may be tempted to increase their medications in order to tolerate a higher activity level or may want to simply remain in bed to stop the pain.

Respect for Pain

As the patient attempts to balance rest and work, pain can be an important protective mechanism that indicates the effectiveness of the balanced program. The nurse needs to assist the patient to identify the source of the joint pain and suggest ways to monitor activities appropriately. The patient needs to understand clearly that pursuing activities despite pain may cause joint damage and that ignoring the symptoms of fatigue may exacerbate the disease process. The patient and family may describe times when one particular event resulted in a swollen knee, or a week of bed rest, or even hospitalization. Ruptured tendons in the hand, ruptured cysts in the knee, or recurrent bursitis all illustrate the vulnerability of joint structures that have been altered by arthritis. The patient needs to see the relationship between *activity* and these joint or systemic symptoms.

The experienced patient with rheumatoid arthritis may notice increasing joint pain that occurs with the *usual* day's activities as a signal of a flare-up of the disease process. Other patients have joint deformities that are readily apparent to the nurse and family members. Destroyed joint space and the loss of articular cartilage may make all activities painful for the damaged joint. Adapted activities or equipment become a critical part of the program, allowing the patient to complete an activity without causing joint pain (e.g., a raised toilet seat to protect a painful knee or hip joint). Other patients may try a new activity or exercise and experience pain. The nurse must reassure and assist the patient to monitor the effects of a *change* in activity level, which may cease to be painful after a few days of adjustment to the new schedule. For the normal individual, the classic example is yard work during a spring or fall weekend, which produces pain in the joints on Monday that carries over to the work week.

Reduction of Effort

Principles of work reduction include (1) avoidance of excessive loads and heavy equipment by incorporating adaptive methods or assistive equipment and (2) incorporation of basic energy conservation principles. All efforts aimed at work reduction or simplification begin with a careful analysis of normal activities and the work environment. Table 3-2 presents a list of questions that may be helpful in teaching patients to analyze their own activities critically.

If the nurse has adaptive equipment available for home instruction, the patient can note the ease or difficulty of rising from a low toilet versus one with a raised seat or getting dressed with or without a protective wrist splint. The patient needs to understand the benefit of an adapted method in reducing pain or making the activity more energy efficient. Once this awareness has been achieved, the patient can become an active partner in working to reduce effort in daily activities. Correct alignment, good posture, and the use of good body mechanics are all part of the reduction of effort. Table 3-3 summarizes some basic strategies for reducing effort and thereby protecting the joints.

Figure 3-1 illustrates the joint protection principle of effort reduc-

Table 3–2   Questions for Activity Analysis

1. How many trips were made between any two points?
2. Could the number of trips be reduced?
3. Could the order of performing different parts of the job be reduced?
4. Are materials and needed equipment within easy reach?
5. Do storage areas contain only the needed materials or are they cluttered with seldom used things?
6. Can any part of this task be omitted or changed and still produce the desired results?
7. Are good body mechanics used in posture, sitting, standing, lifting? How can they be improved?
8. Are both hands used to the best advantage?
9. Would the use of wheels be helpful?
10. Are sitting facilities comfortable and of the proper height?
11. Are the materials prepositioned and ready for use?
12. Is the rate of work too fast?
13. Should someone else do part of the task?

Source: Reprinted with permission from J. L. Melvin, *Rheumatic disease: Occupational therapy and rehabilitation*, 2nd ed. Philadelphia: F. A. Davis, 1982.

Table 3–3   Strategies for Reducing Effort and Protecting the Joints

1. Use the strongest or largest joint possible to perform a task.
    Use the hip to close drawers.
    Use the forearm to close doors.
    Use a shoulder bag instead of a hand bag.
2. Distribute the work load over several joints.
    Use two hands to carry objects.
    Use both arms to lift or reach items.
    Use chairs with arm rests.
3. Use each joint in its most stable and functional position.
    When rising from a chair, keep both feet flat on the floor.
    Stand directly in front of doors to be opened. Avoid twisting the spine.
4. Use good body mechanics.
    Be aware of your posture.
    Avoid unnecessary lifting and carrying.
5. Encourage full and complete joint movement during daily activities.
    Use long, sweeping strokes during housework activities to maintain and increase ROM.
6. Organize your work, use efficient storage, and eliminate unnecessary tasks.

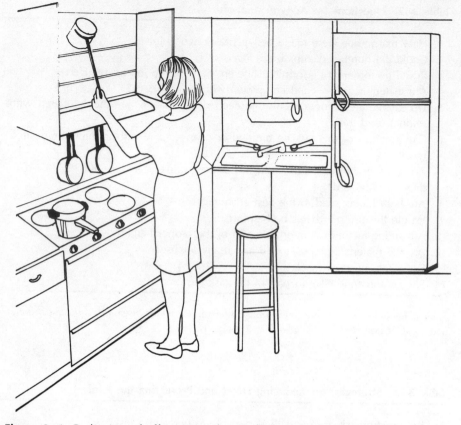

Figure 3–1. Reduction of effort principles applied to the kitchen. Modifications in use: long-handled reacher; built-up faucet handles; cloth loops on refrigerator door; stool to sit on while cooking and washing dishes; double-handled strainer basket; appliances stored within easy reach; and built-up saucepan handles.

tion applied to the kitchen. The stool allows the patient to sit during food preparation, cooking, or dishwashing chores. A long-handled reacher lets the patient reach in order to get items from high shelves. Lazy susans or pullout drawers bring kitchen supplies within easy reach. Cookware is stored on the stove instead of inside cupboards.

Patients often do not realize the many inefficient trips made during common activities or the improper body mechanics employed until a professional observes them completing a task. In the home environment, the nurse is the health professional available to assess these problem areas. The nurse may be able to assist the patient and family to reorganize part of the home during each visit. The same principles illustrated in the kitchen apply.

In the bedroom, for example, are closet shelves within reach and do drawers open easily? Is the bathroom a convenient distance away or would a bedside commode be helpful for day or nighttime use? Are unnecessary clutter or unsafe throw rugs present that could put the patient at risk for a fall? The home visit provides the opportunity to examine all aspects of the home for safety and mobility.

Avoidance of Staying in One Position

Muscles become fatigued in a static position. In addition, prolonged immobility promotes stiffness. When joints are compromised by synovitis or cartilage deterioration, activities such as standing or sitting put additional stresses on the involved joints. Often patients are not aware of the amount of time that is spent performing an activity

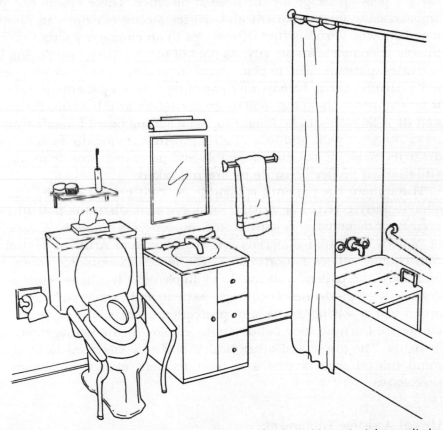

Figure 3–2. Reduction of effort and avoidance of one position principles applied to the bathroom. Modifications in use: built-up faucet handles; built-up toothbrush (or electric toothbrush); suction mat on stool; raised toilet seat; and towels within easy reach.

(e.g., standing at the sink washing dishes, standing in the shower, driving the car, sitting, and watching television). They need to be encouraged to shift positions every 30 to 60 minutes to avoid becoming so stiff that they require assistance to move.

Figure 3-2 illustrates a bathroom that promotes joint protection and lets the patient avoid staying in one position. The shower bench allows the patient to shower sitting down. The raised toilet seat eliminates the need to rise from a low surface. This bathroom should decrease the amount of lower extremity pain that patients experience when standing or getting up from a low position.

Avoidance of Activities That Cannot Be Stopped

Patients can often readily describe to the nurse situations in which they could not walk any further because of joint pain or could not carry a heavy package for the needed distance. These events can be embarrassing for the patient and trigger strong reactions in family members who abruptly find themselves in an emergency situation or unable to complete an activity. As part of the planning and pacing of activities, patients need to plan ahead for activities from which there is no turning back. Anticipatory planning permits patients to take a wheelchair to a shopping mall or grocery store as a backup. Patients and their families can be taught to use a sliding board for safe transfers. The joint pain and loss of strength that frequently accompany arthritis make the patient vulnerable and potentially unsafe in many situations if proper precautions are not taken.

Throughout the patient's education in joint protection, the nurse should provide verbal or written reinforcement when the patient expresses or demonstrates joint protection concepts correctly. A variety of patient education materials are available from Arthritis Foundation chapter offices nationwide. These materials reinforce concepts and allow the patient and family to implement the home care program. These guidelines encourage patient and family participation and problem solving in the joint protection process. The patient and family are learning *new behaviors* to employ in the management of arthritis. The nurse and other health professionals need to keep in mind that change is slow and reinforcement of new behaviors is necessary.

Use of Assistive Equipment

Activities and tasks can be modified in numerous ways to make them less fatiguing and stressful to the involved joints. The assistive devices and equipment used are considered to be joint protection modalities. To be considered effective, any approach must result in pain reduction and preservation of joint integrity by reducing stress on the involved joints. The approach must also successfully assist patients to be more independent in performing activities they would otherwise be unable to do.

The community health nurse can play a significant role in advising patients about assistive equipment and needs to be aware of common items that may be purchased. The nurse also plays an important role in facilitating the acquisition of specific devices in the local community. Equipment needs are therefore carefully evaluated as part of the overall ADL assessment. An occupational therapist should be consulted to prescribe or construct individual pieces of equipment that may be needed to help solve specific ADL problems in the home.

Table 3-4 describes pieces of adaptive equipment that may be used to deal with common problems associated with dressing. Because a wide variety of assistive devices for patients with arthritis are currently on the market, professional prescription of this equipment is essential. If these decisions are left to the family, concerned friends, or the patient, items might be purchased that are difficult to work with, too heavy for swollen joints to use easily, and more frustrating than helpful.

Figure 3-3 illustrates how pieces of adaptive equipment (sockaid),

Table 3–4   Assistive Devices That May Be Used to Solve Common Problems with Dressing

Problem: Inability to Put On or Take Off the Following Articles	Potential Solutions
Bra	Front-opening clothing
Panties	Velcro on clothing
Slacks	Loops on clothing
Shirt	Button hook
Socks	Zipper pull
Shoes	Sockaid
	Long-handled shoe horn
	Dressing stick
	Elastic shoe laces
	Reacher tongs

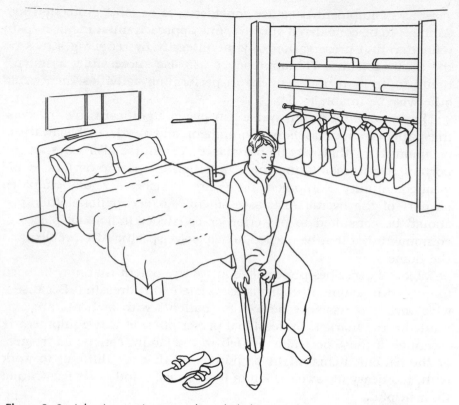

Figure 3–3. Adaptive equipment, adapted clothing, and environmental modifications in the bedroom. Modifications in use: Velcro closures on shoes; cloth loops on socks to put on with a longhandled hook; shelving and storage within easy reach; and sitting to dress.

adapted clothing (Velcro shoes), and an adapted environment (closet shelves, elevated bed, high chair) all come together to create a joint-protecting environment for the patient. Showing illustrations such as this to patients and families will often stimulate multiple ideas for more independent living.

The patient's need for adaptive equipment and assistive devices may fluctuate daily or with major changes in disease status. The patient with rheumatoid arthritis may be more independent when in remission or, on a daily basis, more independent in the afternoon. For example, due to morning stiffness, many patients have difficulty getting on or off the toilet or dressing. These activities are done much more easily later in the morning. The patient may need a raised toilet seat or dressing aids in order to perform ADL independently in the morning. In the afternoon, the patient no longer requires the aids because the morning stiffness has subsided.

Assistive devices may not always be energy-saving for patients with arthritis. Electrical appliances including can openers, knives, and food processors may be too heavy for patients to operate. The buttons may depress with difficulty for patients with thumb deformities. The appliance may be too high once it is resting on the counter to allow the patient with limited shoulder movement to reach and operate it. The patient's home environment and specific disease restrictions need to be carefully evaluated before any piece of equipment is recom-

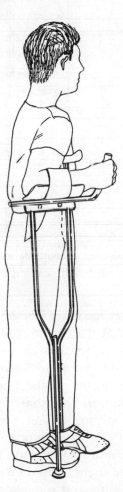

Figure 3—4. Platform crutches. Built-up handles and elbow supports distribute weight more evenly.

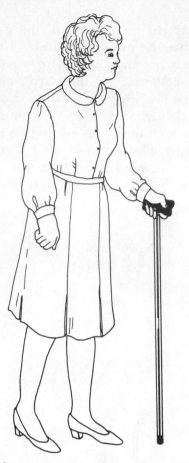

Figure 3–5. Proper fit for a cane. Top of cane is at wrist level when arm hangs relaxed at sides. Elbow is slightly bent while cane is in use.

mended for purchase or use. Assistive devices are prescribed for specific functional problems. A thorough functional evaluation will indicate those areas in which the patient needs assistance.

It is also important for the nurse to keep in mind that adaptive equipment can affect other joints of the body. Canes, crutches, or walkers are common ambulation aids that may be prescribed to protect the joints of the lower extremities. Yet, over time, the use of these devices can adversely affect the wrist, elbow, or shoulder joints.

It is essential that these ambulation aids be accurately measured before use. Patients who use them should be assessed at intervals for signs of nerve pressure or joint and muscle strain. Ambulation aids with built-up handles or elbow supports for weight bearing, such as the platform crutches shown in Figure 3-4, decrease the symptoms of

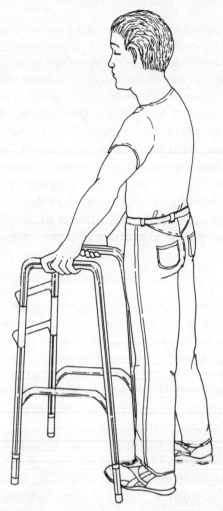

Figure 3–6. Correct height for a walker. Top of walker is at wrist level when arms hang relaxed at sides. Elbows are slightly bent while walker is in use.

arthritis in the wrists and hands. A physical therapist prescribes appropriate ambulatory aids for arthritis patients and should be consulted.

Figure 3-5 illustrates the proper fit for the use of a cane. The fit is correct if the top of the cane is at wrist level when the patient's arm is hanging relaxed at the side. Holding the cane allows the elbow to bend slightly. The correct height for a walker is measured in the same way as for the cane and is illustrated in Figure 3-6. Each assistive device should then be properly introduced to the patient. Patients who need canes, wrist splints, or shoe inserts may have little or no idea what purpose they are designed to serve or how long to use the device without specific instruction from the nurse or therapist.

Simple prescription of an adaptive aid does not, of course, guarantee that the patient will use it. Resistance may be great, especially to highly visible devices such as ambulation aids. The use of the aid may seriously threaten the patient's self-esteem. The reactions of family members and peers are critical. The nurse needs to explore this issue in advance with the patient and family, and seek ways to foster acceptance and compliance. The focus should be placed on independent self-care. The nurse should instruct the patient to monitor general disease symptoms, pain level, and degree of independence in specific tasks while using the equipment over a finite trial period. A positive response will be the most effective stimulus for ongoing use.

Use of Splints

Splints that provide localized rest to a specific joint (e.g., wrist, knee, or ankle) when the arthritis is active are also considered joint protection modalities. As with adaptive aids, thorough assessment of the problem joint and knowledge of the disease process are required before splints are prescribed. During a home visit, the nurse may observe the patient supporting a swollen wrist or painful elbow with the other hand or positioning it on a pillow. The patient may limp noticeably. These are situations that may be improved by the use of splints. The nurse's accurate observations are an important component of the assessment process.

There are numerous commercially available splints for both the upper and lower extremities. Patients may have already purchased elastic supports for problem joints. Patients who are followed in outpatient or inpatient programs may return from a visit with a specific splint fabricated for them by a physical or occupational therapist. These patients frequently do not understand the proper application and use of the splint once they are home. The community health nurse may be the key health care professional in identifying the need for splints and ensuring their correct use at home.

Splints may be prescribed for the stabilization and immobilization of a joint during rest or use. Both the nurse and the patient must be clear about the splint's purpose and use. They should also be clear about the timing for splint use, whether daytime, nighttime, or intermittent. It is important for the nurse to check with the physician or therapist before recommending a splint or assisting a patient to use one at home. If the patient receives a splint from a therapist, checking with the therapist will enable the nurse to reinforce the teaching concerning the correct amount of time for use, as well as the rationale for wearing the splint at home. The nurse can play a valuable role in monitoring both the advantages (pain relief, decreased swelling, support for ADL) and disadvantages (pressure points, increased pain, impaired circulation) of a splinting program in the home. Table 3-5 and Figures 3-7 through 3-19 describe and illustrate specific splints, either custom made or commercially available, that may be used for patients with arthritis.

Table 3–5   Common Splints That May Be Used for Patients with Arthritis

Splint	Rationale	Considerations
1. Soft cervical collar (commercially available)	Protects cervical area. Protects from extreme flexion. Provides pain relief through partial immobilization.	Patient requires ongoing monitoring to avoid muscle weakness.
2. Clavicular strap (commercially available)	Protects weak midback muscles from overuse and maintains normal length of anterior (pectoralis) muscles.	May help maintain posture in patient with early osteoporosis. Flexibility exercises need to accompany the use of this splint.
3. Brown elastic wrist support (commercially available)	Allows limited wrist motion in flexion and extension when wrists are painful. Increases grip strength for hand activities by providing stabilization at the wrist. Decreases symptoms of carpal tunnel syndrome when worn at night.	Custom alterations for optimal fit may be needed. Metal bar can be removed and splint can be worn without it if preferred. Compliance is usually good.

continued

Table 3–5   Common Splints That May Be Used for Patients with Arthritis (*Cont.*)

Splint	Rationale	Considerations
4. Full hand resting splint with C bar (custom made by therapist)	Provides localized rest to involved joints; decreases inflammation and pain. Maintains optimal ROM (combined with strengthening program). Maintains wrist and hand in good alignment.	Consider this splint when patient has persistent synovitis secondary to rheumatoid arthritis. Compliance can be poor due to limited function in splint and degree of immobilization.
5. Ulnar drift positioning (custom made by therapist)	Blocks ulnar drift during pinching and grasping activities to reduce pain and improve function. Repositions fingers in optimal alignment.	Difficult to wear for daily activities because of limited palmar sensation. Compliance may be a concern, especially when multiple splints are suggested.
6. PIP extension splint (custom made by therapist)	Maintains PIP flexion range Decreases or prevents PIP contractures. Useful for swan neck or boutonniere deformities.	Deformities should not be fixed. Can be worn with other kinds of splints.
7. Opponens splint (custom made by therapist)	Relieves pain and increases hand function. This splint is most effective for joint involvement typically seen at the CMC joint in osteoarthritis.	Compliance is good. Splint is comfortable. Useful when hand surgery is not a consideration.
8. Corset (commercially available, usually fit by therapist)	Provide stability by applying counterpressure at abdomen. Restricts movement.	Tolerance of corset in patients with osteoporosis and compression fractures

Table 3–5   Common Splints That May Be Used for Patients with Arthritis (*Cont.*)

Splint	Rationale	Considerations
		of the spine may be a concern.
9. Knee cage (soft) with patella hole (commercially available; usually fit by therapist)	Restricts movement. Protects soft tissue.	Can be difficult for patient to put on without help.
10. Below-knee weight-bearing brace (custom made by orthotist)	Unloads painful ankle by placing weight-bearing at knee joint.	Useful when ankle fusion or total ankle replacement is not an option. Compliance and cost are concerns. Splint is very limiting.
11. Ankle supports can be commercially available or custom made by orthotist—usually fit by therapist.	Restricts motion. Protects soft tissues.	Can be difficult for patient to put on without help.
12. Shoe inserts (custom made by orthotist)	Provides even weight bearing. Redistributes weight-bearing surface to pain-free areas.	Useful in early and later stages of rheumatoid arthritis. Keeps patient ambulatory.
13. Custom-made shoes (commercially available, but usually fit in conjunction with shoe inserts)	Redistributes weight. Relieves pain. Promotes efficient gait.	Useful in early rheumatoid arthritis.

   Splints should be clearly marked to indicate right and left, top and bottom. Once removed, they may be confusing for patients to reapply. The nurse should ask the patient to demonstrate correct removal and reapplication of the splint. Skin irritation is a concern with any splinting device. The patient should be instructed to inspect the skin

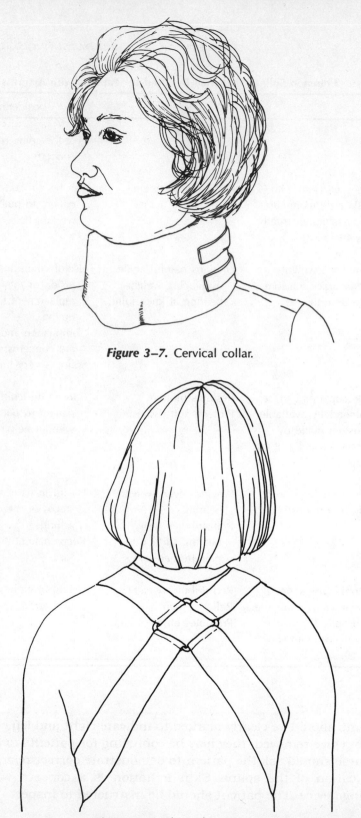

Figure 3–7. Cervical collar.

Figure 3–8. Clavicular strap.

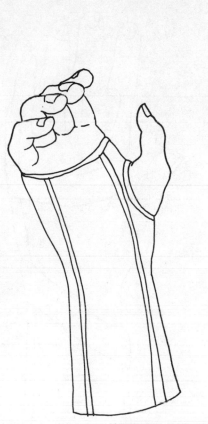
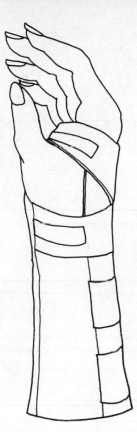

Figure 3–9. Elastic wrist support.

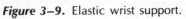
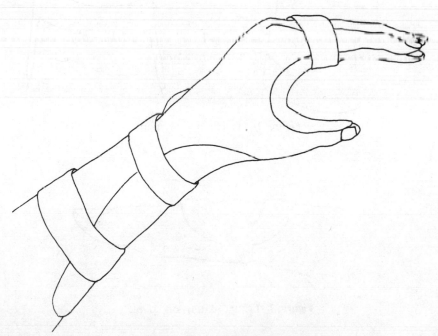

Figure 3–10. Resting hand splint.

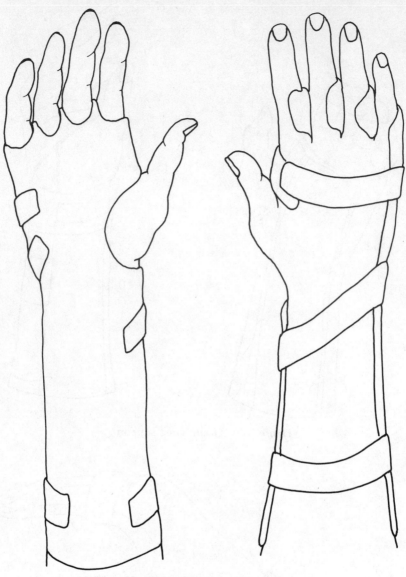

Figure 3–11. Ulnar drift splint.

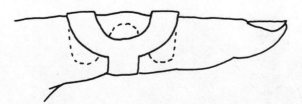

Figure 3–12. PIP extension splint.

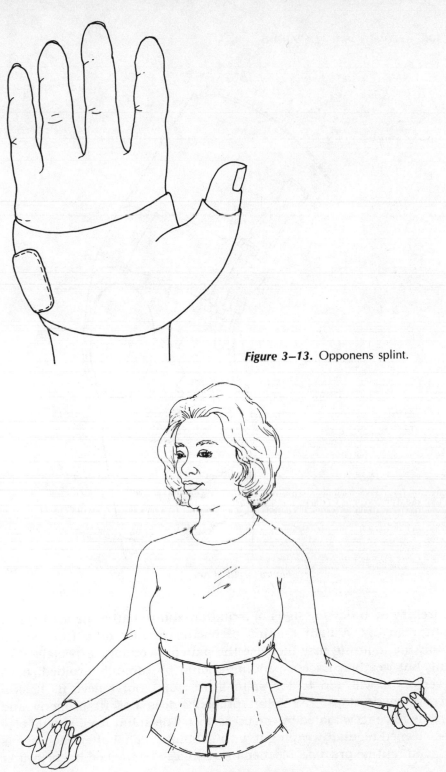

Figure 3–13. Opponens splint.

Figure 3–14. Corset.

99

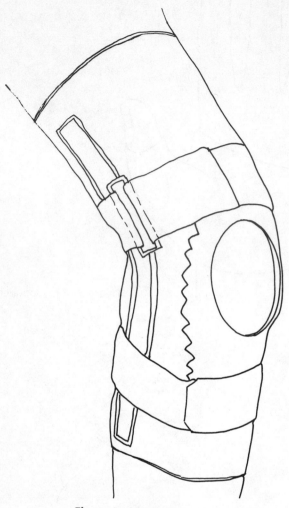

Figure 3–15. Knee cage.

carefully each day for signs of irritation and to bathe the area gently but regularly. A light dusting of talcum powder or a thin cotton stockinette lining may increase the patients comfort, especially during hot weather. Excess padding should be carefully avoided, however, as it will add to the splint's pressure, not relieve it. If skin irritation develops, the splint probably does not fit properly and needs to be reevaluated by the prescriber. The splint itself should also be cleaned regularly. Wiping it with rubbing alcohol after each use is a good routine practice. Most splints can also be washed in cool water

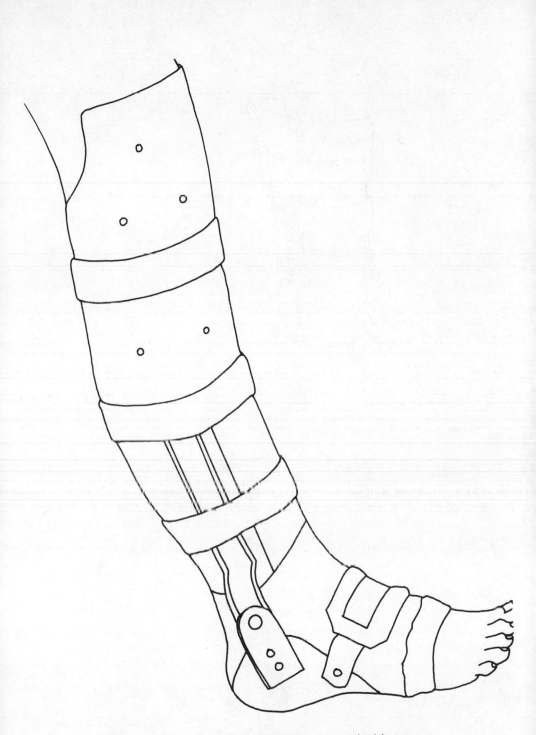

Figure 3–16. Below-knee weight bearing or Tibial brace.

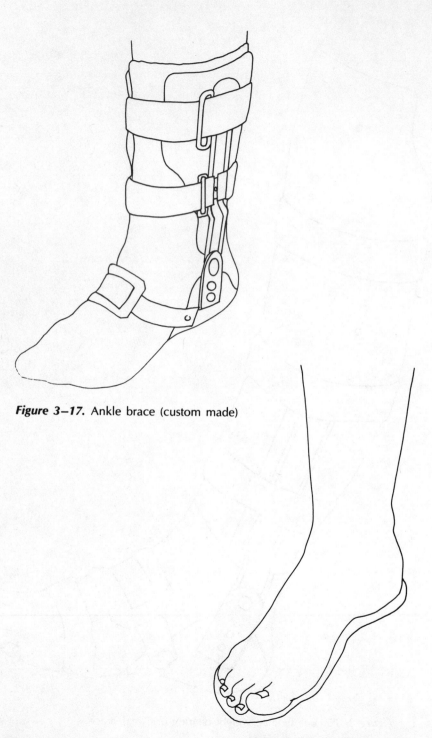

Figure 3-17. Ankle brace (custom made)

Figure 3-18. Shoe insert.

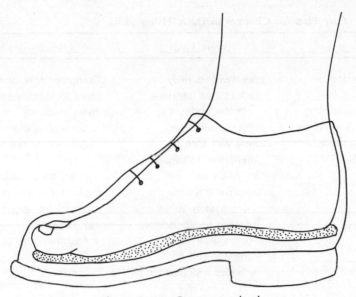

Figure 3-19. Custom-made shoes.

with a mild detergent. Care must be taken to ensure that the splint is completely dry before it is reused.

Table 3-6 summarizes the interventions for changes in daily living skills in care plan format.

EXERCISE FOR RANGE OF MOTION

"Exercise and rest" is a frequently used catch phrase describing the basic elements of the treatment plan. Achieving adequate rest is a major challenge for busy adults, especially during times of increased disease activity. But establishing appropriate home exercise routines is an equal challenge. Too much, too little, or the wrong kind of exercise can all effectively negate any positive outcomes. Routine housework, yard work, and office work may all fatigue the patient significantly and should not be confused with an exercise program.

Range-of-motion (ROM) exercises are exercises in which the patient or the nurse moves the body part through its complete available ROM. These exercises maintain joint mobility for patients with many kinds of arthritis. There are three main forms of ROM exercise, which are described in Table 3-7 and illustrated in Figures 3-20, 3-21, and 3-22.

The terms used to describe ROM exercises, namely, *active* and

Table 3–6 Care Plan for Changes in Daily Living Skills

Nursing Diagnosis	Patient Goal	Interventions
Self-care deficit: bathing/hygiene, dressing/grooming, feeding, or toileting related to the effects of arthritis.	Patient will identify factors that interfere with the ability to provide self-care. Patient will identify alternative strategies for ADLs and use assistive devices appropriately to increase independence. Patient is able to complete self-care activities independently.	1. Complete ADL assessment to identify problem areas involving self-care. Stressful activities Balance of activity and rest Need for adaptive aids 2. Explore alternative methods for accomplishing ADLs. Assistive devices Environmental modifications Consult with occupational therapist regarding assistive device prescription and environmental modifications 3. Assist patient/family in acquiring appropriate assistive devices in the local community. 4. Encourage family to reinforce the ongoing use of assistive devices. 5. Teach family to promote patient independence and provide assistance only as needed.
Knowledge deficit related to joint protection strategies to reduce stress on effected joints.	Patient is knowledgeable about the principles of joint protection. Patient balances activity and rest, and appropriately uses assistive devices, splint or ambulation aids to reduce effort.	1. Clarify joint protection program and adaptive device or splint prescription with occupational therapist. 2. Assist patient to analyze normal activities. 3. Assist patient to develop joint protection strategies to monitor their normal daily activities effectively.

Table 3–6   Care Plan for Changes in Daily Living Skills (*Cont.*)

	4. Reinforce patient teaching about basic disease mechanisms as indicated.
	5. Teach patient to monitor joint symptoms accurately and modify activities in response to pain and inflammation.
	6. Monitor the effectiveness of all joint protection strategies.
	7. Reinforce and support all efforts by the patient to use joint protection strategies.

Table 3–7   Types of ROM Exercise

	Indications for Use	Modalities Employed
1. Passive	Loss of motion without sufficient strength to maintain remaining motion Pain Inability to relax	Therapist Family member
2. Active assistive	Loss of motion Pain Need to maintain and/or increase strength in remaining range	Therapist Family member Pulley Hydrotherapy Wand (cane, broomhandle)
3. Active	Maintain and/or increase ROM Maintain and/or increase strength	Wand Mirror Motivational equipment (exercise videotape)

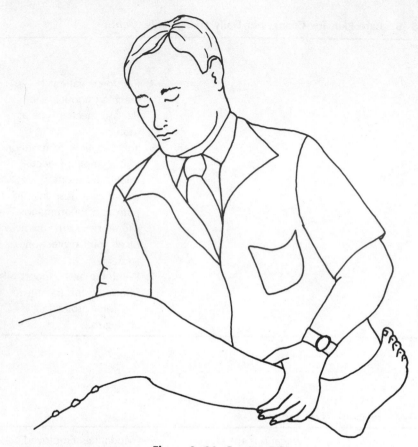

Figure 3–20. Passive ROM.

passive, indicate how the motion should be done but say nothing about the number of repetitions or the amount of force that should be used. If the nurse wants a patient to perform only active exercise, the procedure needs to be carefully demonstrated. Many patients become overzealous and think that if a little is good, more is better, thus causing joint damage.

As with joint protection strategies, it is difficult to provide ongoing rules about exercise. If the joints are warm, reddened, swollen, or painful during an acute disease flare-up, the exercise program may need to be restricted to just one repetition. Further exercise may not be appropriate until the flare-up subsides. Resting splints may be employed during disease flare-ups to prevent contracture and deformity. There may be occasions when *any* movement of the joint is too painful for the patient to tolerate, and exercise may have to be briefly eliminated.

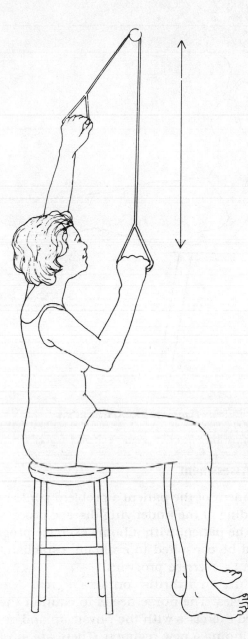

Figure 3–21. Active assistive ROM.

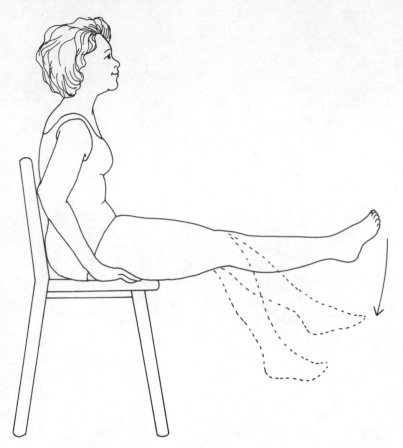

Figure 3–22. Active ROM.

ROM Exercise Assessment

A careful assessment of the patient's problem joints combined with a solid understanding of the underlying disease process will enable the nurse to assist the patient with a home exercise program. A physical therapist should be consulted to evaluate, establish, and modify an individual patient's exercise program.

The lay literature on arthritis contains a great deal of information on specific exercises. The nurse needs to caution the patient to discuss any planned exercises with the physician and/or a physical therapist before beginning a new regimen. There are situations in which exercise is contraindicated. Patients recovering from total joint replacement surgery must take careful precautions while exercising. The presence of fixed or immovable flexion contractures in any joint

Table 3–8   ROM Exercise Assessment

1.   *How joint disease affects ROM*
     Can full ROM be achieved by the individual or is assistance required?
2.   *Type of exercise to use*
     Can the patient tolerate any resistance (weight) during the exercises that
     could be used to strengthen the muscles around the joint?
     How many repetitions can the patient tolerate?
3.   *Time of day*
     Does morning exercise help to relieve the morning stiffness of rheuma-
     toid arthritis?
     Are exercises for the patient with osteoarthritis more beneficial if done
     later in the day, when the joints are more mobile?
     What is the optimal time of day for exercise, considering the patient's
     work and home schedule?
4.   *Follow-up*
     Who will be responsible for monitoring the exercise program?
     What plans are made for increasing or decreasing the number of
     repetitions and adding resistance if the patient shows improvement?

contraindicates the use of ROM exercise. The sound of creaking or crepitus in the joint as bone moves against bone can be frightening to both the patient and the nurse. Consultation with a physical therapist ensures patient safety and compliance with the recommended type and duration of exercise. Table 3-8 summarizes some basic points to consider in ROM exercise assessment.

An essential ingredient of all exercise programs is follow-up. Because the nurse is able to enter the home environment, the duration, benefits, problems, and progress with the exercise program can be noted, evaluated, and documented for the family, physician, or therapist. Patients may stay at a comfortable level of activity and exercise unless the nurse facilitates an increase in the level of the program. Charts and graphs help record the number and duration of exercises for the nurse and the patient, and can be motivators for completing a program.

How Much Exercise and How Often?

The duration of pain is usually a good guide for prescribing exercise. Pain or discomfort resulting from the exercise should not last for more than an hour afterward. If joint pain lasts for several hours or if the patient feels excessive joint discomfort the next day, the exercises were too stressful and should be reduced. When inflammation is present, anti-inflammatory measures must be taken in addition to the ROM exercises.

Melvin (1982) states: "There is no hard and fast rule regarding the number of repetitions necessary to maintain or increase mobility. Some patients, for example, those with stable, chronic conditions, may need to perform only one complete ROM daily for maintenance, while patients in an acute or subacute phase (when there is more periarticular swelling and less physical activity) may need to perform more complete ROMs per day" (p. 385). The only certainty in a chronic disease such as rheumatoid arthritis is its *uncertainty*. An exercise program requires monitoring by the health professional for maximum benefit.

EXERCISE FOR MUSCLE STRENGTH AND ENDURANCE

Exercise for strengthening muscles takes two forms: isometric and isotonic. Community health nurses may be most familiar with isometric quadriceps or gluteal set exercises. Isometric exercises are useful for patients with arthritis because the muscle contracts without moving the painful joint through its range of motion.

A program of isometric exercises can be prescribed for individual joints. The procedure includes having the patient contract the specific muscle as tightly as possible without moving the joint, hold for about 6 seconds, and then relax for 6 seconds. The procedure is performed for the prescribed number of repetitions. A physical therapist will prescribe this program for individual patients. Figures 3-23A and 3-23B illustrate two applications of isometric exercise.

Isotonic exercises allow for a definite grading of resistance (weights) during the exercise. The type of resistance can vary from very gentle manual pressure to the application of heavy weights. This particular part of the exercise program must be prescribed and monitored by a physical therapist, as it is specific to individual patients. The nurse should remind patients not to initiate any changes in their exercise regimen without consulting with the physical therapist. The decision to implement such a program is based on several factors. The extent of disease involvement in individual joints is crucial, as is the extent of systemic disease. How the exercise program will fit into a patient's daily routine is another important consideration. Table 3-9 summarizes basic information about the use of strengthening exercise.

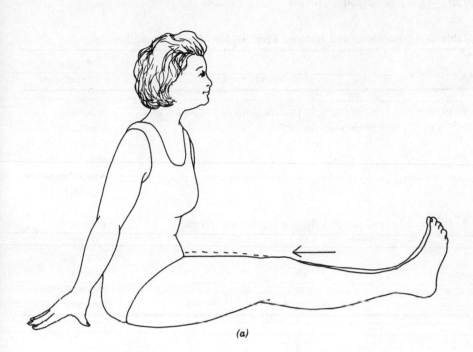

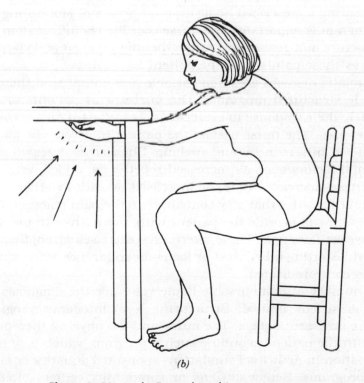

Figure 3–23. (a, b) Examples of isometric exercise.

Table 3–9   Isometric and Isotonic Exercise for Muscle Strengthening

	Indications for Use	Modalities Employed
1. Isometric	Loss of strength, but movement is painful or potentially damaging.	Sandbags Therapist Others Self Any immovable object
2. Isotonic	Loss of strength, but significant motion is preserved.	Therapist Others Sandbags Pulleys Elastic rope Barbells

The nurse can offer patients significant assistance in successfully implementing a prescribed home exercise program. Monitoring of the total program is important. The nurse coordinates information about the structure and goals of the strengthening regimen and clarifies or reinforces these points with the patient as needed.

Rheumatic diseases are often variable and do not lend themselves to tightly structured programs. The nurse helps patients to assess accurately their response to exercise. Increased pain may accompany new exercises. The nurse assists the patient to assess the joints for signs of warmth, redness, and swelling. She also analyzes other environmental factors such as increased repetitions, added weight with the exercise, increased time, or increased activity in other work or household activities that may contribute to the pain reaction. A flexible program will provide the patient with alternatives to use during mild disease flare-ups. These alternative exercises strengthen some joints while letting others rest or focus on endurance when strengthening is contraindicated.

The number of reimbursable home visits for the diagnosis of arthritis is strictly limited. Structuring a maintenance program is therefore an essential task. The nurse and the physical therapist can work with the patient to outline such a program, which may include participation in Arthritis Foundation—sponsored aquatics or land exercise programs. Senior citizens or community centers often have programs to provide exercise that is safe and enjoyable for many persons. The nurse can assist the patient and family to explore resources in the local community, as well as devise strategies to overcome common barriers to adherence such as transportation, cost, and scheduling. Table 3-10 summarizes the basic concerns about changes in mobility in a care plan format.

Table 3-10   Care Plan for Changes in Mobility

Nursing Diagnosis	Patient Goal	Interventions
Impaired physical mobility related to pain and restricted joint motion.	Patient will identify factors that interfere with mobility. Patient will maintain full ROM in body joints through appropriate use of active and passive exercise. Patient will adjust exercise regimen as needed in response to fluctuating disease activity.	1. Complete ROM and exercise assesment including: Effects of arthritis on joint ROM Current exercise regimen/tolerance and compliance 2. Clarify exercise prescription with physical therapist and reinforce teaching as needed. Type of exercise Amount of weight or resistance Number of repetitions Modifications for disease flare-ups 3. Reinforce importance of correct posture and joint alignment. 4. Teach patient respect for pain.
Activity intolerance related to decreased strength and endurance.	Patient will establish an activity/rest pattern consistent with joint limitations. Patient will successfully integrate an exercise program into the daily routine.	1. Consult with physical therapist. 2. Assess patient's level of fatigue and its pattern. 3. Explore correct timing for exercise in patient's daily life.

continued

Table 3–10 Care Plan for Changes in Mobility (*Cont.*)

Nursing Diagnosis	Patient Goal	Interventions
	Patient will increase strength and endurance.	4. Reinforce patient teaching concerning isometric and isotonic exercise as needed. 5. Monitor patient's progress in regard to overall program goals. 6. Assess the response of individual joints to the exercise regimen. 7. Provide regular support and reinforcement to the patient and family. 8. Explore community resources for ongoing exercise involvement.

CASE STUDIES

1. Maria Palmero is a 32-year-old married woman who was diagnosed with rheumatoid arthritis 6 years ago. She has four children between the ages of 3 and 11. The family has limited financial resources and lives on the top floor of a garden apartment building with laundry facilities in the basement. Mrs. Palmero's husband is supportive but works long hours at his job and is rarely at home. The family has many family members and friends in the area, and Mr. Palmero likes to socialize and invite people for meals on weekends.

   Mrs. Palmero has suffered several disease flare-ups in the last few years and does not respond to NSAIDs. She is being followed in the early stages of a gold therapy protocol. Mrs. Palmero confides that she is constantly tired and that her joints seem to hurt all the time, especially in her hands and wrists. When questioned about her exercise routine, she replies, "Exercise? I get all I can take running after these kids! Do you know how much energy a 3-year-old has?" Mrs. Palmero does not use any assistive devices or adaptive aids and does not appear to be familiar with the principles of joint protection.

   1. What data do you need to obtain as part of your ADL and exercise assessment?
   2. What strengths do you identify in Mrs. Palmero's current situation? What specific limitations?

3. What assistive devices, adaptive aids, or environmental modifications might be explored to reduce the effort involved in Mrs. Palmero's daily routine?

4. What specific recommendations could you make to assist her in better balancing activity and rest?

5. What type and amount of exercise might be beneficial to her?

2. John Jefferson is a 75-year-old man with long-standing osteoarthritis in his spine, hips, and knees. He lives alone in a small, one-story house. His general appearance is thin and frail, and he readily admits that he lacks energy and sleeps a lot. Mr. Jefferson has no family or friends in the area and admits that he spends virtually all of his time alone. He has gradually stopped his involvement with his church and the local senior citizens group.

Total joint replacement was recommended to Mr. Jefferson 10 years ago, but he always refused. He is now quite incapacitated. He receives meals on wheels, and a local woman provides basic cleaning and shopping services once a week. He has never followed a formal exercise program and "protects" his joints by remaining immobile in his reclining chair whenever he has a bad day. On most days he neither prepares meals for himself nor dresses.

1. What further assessment data would be useful in helping to plan Mr. Jefferson's care?

2. What goals involving ADLs and mobility would be appropriate for Mr. Jefferson, considering his disease status and age?

3. What advantages are present in his situation to facilitate their accomplishment? What limitations must be overcome?

4. Are there any assistive devices, adaptive aids, or environmental modifications that might be useful in meeting these patient goals?

5. What strategies might be used to begin to deal with Mr. Jefferson's fatigue and muscle weakness? What type of exercise program might be helpful and acceptable?

PATIENT EDUCATION MATERIALS

Arthritis Society. (1982). *Adjusting to rheumatoid arthritis and how to conserve energy and protect joints.* The Arthritis Society, 920 Yonge St., Suite 420, Toronto, Ontario M4W 3J7, Canada.

Clearinghouse. (1984). *Exercise for older Americans.* National Health Information Clearinghouse, Box 1133, Washington, DC 20013-1133.

Haviland, N., Jette, A. M., & Duff, I. F. (1982). *Joint protection for osteoar-thritis.* University of Michigan Medical Campus, Media Library—R-4440, Kresge 1, Box 56, Ann Arbor, MI 48109.

Haviland, N., Kamil-Miller, L., & Silwa, J. (1978). *A workbook for consumers with rheumatoid arthritis: Joint protection principles.* American Occupational Therapy Association, Inc., 1383 Piccard Dr., Suite 300, Rockville, MD 20850.

Jetter, J., & Kadlec, N. (1985). *The arthritis book of water exercise.* Holt, Rinehart & Winston, 383 Madison Ave., New York, NY 10017.

Kantz, C. (1981). *Joint protection for rheumatoid arthritis.* Rosalind Russell Arthritis Center, University of California—San Francisco, 1442 Fifth Ave., San Francisco, CA 94143.

Sargent, J. V. (1982). *An easier way: Handbook for the elderly and handi-capped.* Walker & Company, 720 Fifth Ave., New York, NY 10019.

Wiggins, P., Freeman, L., & Collier, M. (1983). *Arthritis—Fighting the wear and tear—a patient guide to self-management.* Medical University of South Carolina, Division of Rheumatology and Immunology, 171 Ashley Ave., Charleston, SC 29425.

AUDIOVISUAL MATERIALS

Arthritis Foundation. (1979). *Rheumatoid arthritis: Rest and exercise.* Dallas Area Hospital Television Services, University of Texas Health Science Center, 5323 Harry Hines Blvd., Dallas, TX 75235.

Dillingham, P. (1983). *Arthritis therapy exercise.* International Gerontology Consultants, 4723 Summerhill Rd., Las Vegas, NV 89121.

Harlowe, D., & Yu, P. B. (1984). *The ROM dance: A range of motion exercise and relaxation program.* Friends of WHA-TV—Program Marketing, 821 University Ave., Madison, WI 53706.

Karl•Lorimar. (1984). *Jane Powell's fight back with fitness.* Karl•Lorimar Home Video, Inc., 17942 Cowan, Irvine, CA 92714.

Mini Productions. (1980). *Therapy in motion.* MTI Teleprograms, Inc., 3710 Commercial Ave., Northbrook, IL 60062.

Wickersham, B. (1982). *Exercises for people with arthritis.* Southwest Arthritis Center, 2033 E. Speedway, Tucson, AZ 85719.

BIBLIOGRAPHY

Banwell B. F. (1984). Exercise and mobility in arthritis. In D. Hawley, ed., *Arthritis: Impact on people* (pp. 80–146). Philadelphia: W. B. Saunders.

Cordery, J. C. (1965). Joint protection: A responsibility of the occupational therapist. *American Journal of Occupational Therapy, 19,* 285–289.

Feinberg, J., & Brandt, K. D. (1981). Use of resting splints by patients with rheumatoid arthritis. *American Journal of Occupational Therapy, 35*(3), 173–178.

Furst, G. P., Gerber, L. H., Smith, C. C., Fisher, S., & Shullman, B. (1987). A program for improving energy conservation behaviors in adults with rheumatoid arthritis. *American Journal of Occupational Therapy, 41,* 102–111.

Halpern, A. A. (1984). *Exercise and physical therapy.* Philadelphia: George F. Stickley.

Krewer, S. (1981). *The arthritis exercise book.* New York: Simon & Schuster.

Lorig, K., & Fries, J. F. (1986). *The arthritis helpbook.* Reading, Mass.: Addison-Wesley.

Machover, S., & Sapecky, A. J. (1966). Effect of isometric exercise on the quadriceps muscle in patients with rheumtoid arthritis. *Archives of Physical Medicine and Rehabilitation, 47,* 737–741.

McDuffie, F. C., & Boutaugh, M. (1985). Pool exercise programs for people with arthritis. *Clinical Rheumatology in Practice, 3*(4), 168–169.

Melvin, J. L. (1982). *Rheumatic disease: Occupational therapy and rehabilitation,* 2nd ed. Philadelphia: F. A. Davis.

Pedretti, L. W. (1985). Activities of daily living. In L. W. Pedretti, ed., *Occupational therapy: Practice skills for physical dysfunction,* 2nd ed. (pp. 141–170). St. Louis: C. V. Mosby.

Porter, S. F., Dapper, M. J., & Foran, C. (1980). Hand splints. *American Journal of Nursing, 80*(2), 276–278.

Rosenberg, A. L. (1979). *Living with your arthritis: A home program for arthritis management.* New York: Arco.

Silwa, J. (1982). Performance objectives for joint protection instruction. In J. L. Melvin, ed. *Rheumatic disease: Occupational therapy and rehabilitation,* pp. 352–353.

Trombley, C. A., & Scott, A. D. (1977). Home evaluation. In C. A Trombley & A. D. Scott (eds.), *Occupational therapy for physical dysfunction* (pp. 399–406). Baltimore: Williams & Wilkins.

Wickersham, B. A. (1984). The exercise program. In G. K. Riggs & E. P. Gall (eds.), *Rheumatic disease: Rehabilitation and management.* (pp. 115–129). Boston: Butterworth.

Wilske, K. R. (1980). *Therapeutic program for the patient with arthritis,* 3rd ed. Seattle: Mason Clinic.

4

Changes in Sexuality

Sarah A. Liddle
Judith K. Sands

Sexuality is an integral portion of our daily lives. Not limited to the functioning of the male and female genitalia, sexuality influences the physiologic, psychologic, and sociologic components of a person's being. This holistic perspective on sexuality has gradually emerged as American society has abandoned the traditionally expressed view that the sole purpose of sexuality is reproduction.

The unfolding of our awareness that sexuality holds a central position in human existence has created a serious dilemma for health care providers. If sexual health is viewed as an important aspect of the patient's overall health and personality, it must be considered in assessment and care planning. Health professionals have not, however, traditionally considered sexuality to be an essential aspect of overall patient care. Therefore, both medicine and nursing have often avoided the entire issue of the patient's sexual health. General discomfort, plus the feeling of being ill prepared to deal with this sensitive topic, have contributed to a basic avoidance of sexuality as a legitimate area of concern and intervention. The acute care setting, by its nature, has also supported this general avoidance of sexuality with its focus on life-and-death issues. The community setting has also commonly ignored the topic of sexuality, as caregivers' belief that they are guests in the patient's home makes it difficult or inappropriate to approach the subject. The topic of sexuality, therefore, too often remained and remains unvoiced.

Nursing professionals in all settings must increase their skill and comfort in dealing with problems related to sexuality. We are only beginning to realize the extent to which health problems of all types affect an individual's sexual health. Nurses must be alert to that effect; open and willing to address sexual issues with patients; and knowledgeable about the resources for information and assistance available in the community. This chapter addresses the impact that arthritis may have on an individual's sexual health and discusses intervention strategies that may be used to assist patients who are experiencing sexual difficulties.

ARTHRITIS AND SEXUALITY

The diagnosis of arthritis affects an individual's sexuality in both general and specific ways. Although effective treatment is available, arthritis is a chronic disease with no potential for cure. During an episode of acute temporary illness, individuals in our society are permitted and encouraged to put aside active sexual behavior for a time and focus their mental and physical energy on the task of getting well. Individuals resume their previous pattern of functioning as the illness resolves. Chronic illness, however, does not allow for this natural resolution process. Instead, at the end of an acute episode, chronically ill individuals are still challenged to function successfully in their traditional environment within the limits of their disabilities. With arthritis patients, the nature and scope of those disabilities may include changes in body image, comfort, role performance, and autonomy. All of these affect some aspect of sexuality and require patients to make significant adaptive changes if they are to maintain sexual identity and health. In addition, these changes do not occur in a vacuum. They significantly affect the patient's relationships with the spouse, family, and significant others. Sexual relationships are common victims.

The available research that addresses sexuality in arthritis reinforces the importance of interventions aimed at sexual health. A survey conducted by the Moss Rehabilitation Hospital in Philadelphia explored the effect of arthritis on the individual's sexual life (Johnson, 1975). The study found that:

1. 53% of the patients reported that they had altered their sexual activity.
2. 57% of the patients reported that they had experienced decreased interest.
3. 54% of the patients reported that they had experienced decreased satisfaction.
4. 78% of the patients reported a decrease in the frequency of sexual relations.
5. 61% of the patients reported that they had altered their sexual interaction to some degree.

Elst (1984), Ferguson and Figley (1979), and Yoshino and Uchida (1981) all report findings that support the conclusion that arthritis affects sexuality in significant and diverse ways.

Common Areas of Concern

Comfort

Joint pain and stiffness are daily factors in the lives of persons with arthritis. These alterations in comfort can affect sexuality in several ways. The simple fact that pain is present on a regular basis can significantly decrease the individual's interest in sexual activity. The task of dealing with pain consumes both time and energy. The arthritis patient is frequently chronically fatigued and may lack the energy for sexual functioning. The physical act of intercourse may be difficult, due in part to pain, particularly when the hip joint is involved. Pain and stiffness in the hands, arms, and mandibular joints may interrupt the individual's ability and desire to engage in even the most simple forms of intimacy such as touching, hugging, and kissing.

The presence of pain also has a significant potential impact on a caring sexual partner, which is important to acknowledge. Facial or verbal expressions of discomfort may cause partners to suppress their own desire for sexual contact out of fear of inflicting pain or of appearing selfish and uncaring when expressing their desire for sexual intimacy. Obviously this suppression of sexuality can have extremely detrimental effects on the relationship. Sexual contact is broken off, and the free communication of thoughts and desires is impaired.

Body Image

Body image represents an integration of the person's feelings about his or her body and its functions and the feedback that is received about how others view it. A positive body image is one of the important components of sexual health. The joint limitations and physical changes that frequently accompany arthritis may have a negative effect on body image. Visible changes such as the common deformities of the hands and feet, gait changes, abnormalities caused by hip and knee involvement, and surgical scars can be particularly troublesome. Our societal preoccupation with physical attractiveness, youth, beauty, and fitness makes physical changes that limit mobility of particular concern.

The importance of these body changes will vary significantly from individual to individual, but all arthritis patients must make an adaptation to them. When joint changes are interpreted as an indication that the patient is less masculine or feminine, this belief affects sexual health and functioning. Patients may be worried about becoming less attractive as sexual partners. In this context, they are likely to interpret any lessening of sexual overtures or activity on the part of the spouse or sexual partner as rejection, no matter what the real reason may be.

Role Function

The multiple roles that we play in daily living and our functioning in those roles are an important part of the development and maintenance of body image and self esteem. Some of these roles are defined by gender identity, helping to establish masculine and feminine images, and therefore are a part of sexuality. Changes in role performance necessitated by disease processes are particularly devastating when they affect the performance of basic family and social roles that existed in the predisease state.

Arthritis affects an individual's performance in the most basic ways, threatening independence and competence in roles such as breadwinner, housewife, mother/father, spouse, and lover. Loss of competencies in these roles may seriously disturb the individual's self concept, especially when a job change or loss of employment results. The inability to fulfill a socially designated role successfully can mortally wound the patient's self-image as a worthwhile man or woman. The implications for the individual's sexual image may be devastating.

Autonomy

The unpredictability of the course of arthritis adds special stresses to the patient's overall disease adaptation. The pattern of exacerbation and remission, which may occasionally involve hospitalization, keeps the patient off balance. The need to follow a treatment regimen involving daily exercise and medication also challenges the patient's control. Even the assistive devices that are an essential part of joint protection programs serve to underscore the patient's increasing dependence on things and on other persons. Financial burdens may force the patient to seek or use outside support that has never been previously considered. The patient's autonomy is significantly threatened. Spiraling dependence demands that the patient continuously readjust body image, self-concept, and role expectations, further enhancing the burdening effects of change.

NURSING MANAGEMENT

Nurses are in a unique position to intervene successfully with patients who have problems or concerns involving their sexuality. Nurses spend more time with patients than do other members of the health care team and are often the persons with whom the patient is most comfortable. Nurses routinely assist individuals with basic physical processes and are accorded a degree of intimacy that few other professionals achieve. This special relationship can be effectively used to deal with the sensitive issues of sexuality.

Nurses who are knowledgeable about sexuality and comfortable enough with the topic to provide basic information, counseling, or referral to appropriate community resources can make a significant contribution to their patients' well-being. Even if a nurse does not feel that she has sufficient knowledge to give direct counseling, she can still provide significant service to the patient by simply incorporating sexual assessment into the total assessment process, listening as the patient expresses concerns, and providing the patient with access to other informational resources.

Every nurse who works with arthritis patients should be familiar with the Arthritis Foundation's excellent pamphlet entitled "Living and Loving."* Providing a copy ensures that the patient at least has access to sound information about sexuality. Katz (1986) found that 48% of arthritis patients prefer to receive sexual advice from written material. Another 37% prefer this advice to come directly from a health professional. If patients prefer to discuss their sexual concerns with the nurse, the pamphlet has at least served to legitimize sex as an acceptable topic for discussion. If the patient's needs are beyond the nurse's area of expertise, an appropriate referral can be initiated.

Assessment of Sexual Health

The 1975 World Health Organization's definition of sexual health reflects the complexity of the concept of sexuality. It states that "sexual health is the integration of the somatic, emotional, intellectual, and social aspects of sexual beings, in ways that are positively enriching and that enhance personality, communication and love." This definition clearly supports the idea that sexuality affects or is a part of virtually every aspect of an individual's life. This holistic perspective can make the idea of sexual assessment rather daunting. Where would you begin and how would you know what should be included? In reality, aspects of sexuality are already being assessed as nurses explore with patients the impact of their disease process on their patterns of daily living. Unfortunately, the area of assessment that is most commonly overlooked or avoided by nurses is that which deals

---

* Copies can be obtained through local chapters of the Arthritis Foundation.

directly with the sexual practices and concerns of the patient.

Before making any attempt to intervene with patients about sexual concerns, it is essential that the nurse first explore her own value system concerning sexuality and consider its impact on her thinking and interventions. Nurses cannot afford to adopt a limited moralistic position if they are to be of assistance to their patients. A nurse who communicates that she is opposed to the very idea of alternatives in sexual expression eliminates any possibility of meaningful problem solving with the patient.

Sexual health assessment focuses on gathering data in four general areas. These areas will now be discussed.

Sexual Functioning and Practices Before Illness. Information in the area of sexual functioning and practices before the patient's illness provides a base from which to begin to plan interventions. No assumptions should be made about the type or frequency of sexual activity in which the patient engages or even about whether the patient is sexually active. Gathering data about sexual functioning means accepting the possibility of patient homosexuality or of married couples who practice extended abstinence.

The nature, frequency, and types of sexual practices engaged in and the patient's level of enjoyment and satisfaction need to be explored. Patients with negative or indifferent past sexual histories will obviously respond differently to the changes necessitated by the disease process than those with a history of satisfying and pleasurable sexual relationships. This information will lay the groundwork for decisions concerning interventions.

Physical Effects of the Illness or Its Treatment. Although arthritis rarely has a direct effect on the sexual organs or their functioning, it obviously has multiple physical effects on sexuality. Pain, joint and muscle stiffness, contractures, and fatigue all directly affect the physical ability of patients to engage in their normal sexual activities. These effects need to be specifically addressed in the assessment process.

Patient Perceptions of and Response to the Illness. Because sexuality affects so many aspects of an individual's lifestyle, it is important to consider and explore many areas in order to obtain an accurate picture of the effects of arthritis on the individual's sexuality. Body image, role function changes, perceptions of masculinity and femininity, and libido are all important areas to consider. It is obvious that not all of them can be explored in depth at one sitting. This is especially true because the impact of arthritis in some of these areas may not be clear, conscious, or apparent to the patient and will be acknowledged only through ongoing work with the nurse.

Response of the Spouse or Sexual Partner to the Illness. A disease process such as arthritis does not affect the patient in isolation from his or her social network. Instead, each change that occurs in response to the disease affects the entire family unit. The sexual relationship is uniquely vulnerable. A partner's illness or disability may become a stimulus for special closeness and sensitivity between two people, or it may act as a stressor that drives a wedge between the partners and erodes the relationship.

Open sexual communication between two partners cannot be assumed. Where optimal communication does not already exist, the stress imposed by the limitations of arthritis can significantly weaken the relationship. The healthy partner may withdraw from sexual activity out of fear of causing pain, but this action may be interpreted by the patient as rejection rather than loving concern. The patient's natural concerns over physical attractiveness and the ability to satisfy the partner may become overwhelming. Whatever the initial motives, the end result can be a downward spiral of resentment, isolation, and rejection on the part of both partners. The spouse or partner must be included in the assessment phase to achieve even minimal insight into the nature of the relationship.

Strategies for Assessment

Questions about disease-related changes in sexual functioning are most easily dealt with by directly incorporating them into the broader ADL assessment. This indicates clearly that sexuality is considered to be one of the functions of daily living and does not single it out for special consideration. The University of Michigan Arthritis Center suggests simply asking the patient "Has your disease caused a change in your sexual functioning?" as a means of initiating the assessment of sexuality (Figley, Ferguson, Bole, & Kay, 1980). If the answer is "yes," the follow-up question "Is that a concern for you?" is appropriate. The remainder of the assessment is left as an open-ended interview. Extensive or detailed forms impose an impersonality on the process that does not support the sensitive nature of the assessment. The major advantage of this approach is the fact that it allows the patient to define the problem and to control further exploration of the subject.

Table 4–1   Approaches to Sexual Assessment

1. Has your arthritis interfered with your being a (mother, wife, father, husband)?	1. What can you do sexually?
2. Has your arthritis changed the way you feel about yourself as a (man, woman)?	2. What can't you do sexually?
3. Has your arthritis changed your ability to function sexually?	3. What do you want to do sexually?
N.F. Woods (1984)	S.A. Liddle

Source: A portion of this table has been reproduced by permission from Nancy Fugate Woods: *Human Sexuality in Health and Illness*, 3rd ed. St. Louis: C. V. Mosby Co., 1984, p. 88.

There is no need for the sexual assessment to be a lengthly process, although the data base will certainly expand if a nurse works with a patient over time. Table 4-1 contains two assessment tools that use very different approaches to the patient, yet each contains only three questions. The Woods approach (1984) is indirect and the Liddle approach is direct, but both seek to elicit comparable types of information. The nurse may decide which one to use based on her own comfort with the style of the questions. Even though the actual questions are few and brief, it is essential that sufficient time be allotted to the assessment process for more detailed exploration of the patient's response. Skill in interviewing will, of course, facilitate the process, but the major requirements on the part of the nurse are sensitivity and the ability to listen empathically in order to understand the problem from the patient's perspective.

Privacy is essential, and the failure to provide it clearly communicates to the patient both a lack of respect and a lack of seriousness about discussing sexual issues. This is especially important in a home environment, where the nurse may need to request the patient to establish the conditions of privacy.

Confidentiality goes hand in hand with privacy and may be of real concern to the patient and partner. Documentation is an essential aspect of professional care, but this does not mean that specific details of the assessment or interventions need to be recorded. The nurse may simply document that sexual concerns have been discussed and indicate the patient teaching or referrals that were made. Table 4-2 summarizes some practical suggestions and guidelines to be followed by the nurse while completing a sexual assessment.

Table 4–2 General Guidelines for Conducting an Interview Regarding Sexuality

Do	Don't
1. Obtain information about all need areas.	1. Focus only on sexuality.
2. Provide privacy.	2. Obtain information when others are present or take copious notes.
3. Strive for an unhurried atmosphere.	3. Check your watch, tap your foot.
4. Maintain an attitude that is frank, open, warm, objective, empathetic.	4. Project discomfort, become defensive.
5. Use nondirective techniques when possible.	5. Ask many direct questions.
6. Have a prepared introduction to state purpose of interview.	6. Be vague about the purpose of the interview.
7. Use appropriate vocabulary.	7. Use street terms.
8. "Check out" words to ensure patient understands.	8. Assume the patient understands what you're saying.
9. Adjust the order of questions according to client's needs.	9. Follow a rigid format.
10. Give client time to think and answer questions.	10. Answer questions for client.
11. Recognize signs of anxiety.	11. Focus on getting information without recognizing patient feeling.
12. Give permission not to do something.	12. Have preset expectations of the patient's sexual activity.
13. Listen in an interested but matter-of-fact way.	13. Overreact or underreact.
14. Identify your attitudes, values, beliefs, and feelings.	14. Project your concerns or problems on to the patient.
15. Identify significant others.	15. Assume that no one else is involved in the patient/client's sexual concerns.
16. Identify philosophical religious beliefs of patient/client.	16. Inflict your moral judgments on the patient.
17. Acknowledge when you don't have an answer to a question.	17. Pretend you know when you don't.

Source: Reprinted with permission from R. Hogan, *Human sexuality—a nursing perspective.* East Norwalk, Conn: Appleton & Lange, 1985.

Nursing Interventions

A number of strategies can be suggested to the arthritis patient to deal with the typical problems that affect sexual activity. Probably the most important nursing intervention, however, is the sexual assessment. This assessment communicates to the patient that it is appropriate to be concerned over the impact of arthritis on sexual functioning and to discuss those concerns with the nurse. Routine interventions include information sharing, communication, and symptom management.

Information Sharing

Americans are often sadly uninformed about the nature of male and female sexual functioning. Partial ignorance in this area may be compounded by misinformation concerning the effects of arthritis and its treatment on sexuality. Obviously, both the patient and the partner need specific information that addresses any and all of the myths, questions, and misconceptions that they may have. Verbalizing fears and concerns may be a successful intervention in itself. Simply hearing a nursing professional address issues related to sexuality may be a sufficient intervention in certain situations.

Communication

Reestablishing or improving communication with the partner is the first step in dealing with problems in a sexual relationship. Open and effective communication has been consistently shown to enhance sexual functioning and is a basic tool of sex therapy. Because of the numerous ways in which arthritis can negatively affect a sexual relationship, the partners need to be able to talk openly about their sexual needs and to establish both what is satisfying and pleasurable and what is uncomfortable. This type of discussion may not come easily or naturally to couples who may have fallen into a pattern of prolonged abstinence. When communication is acknowledged as a problem, the nurse can offer significant assistance by speaking with both partners in order to initiate the communication process and by reminding the couple of the importance of setting aside time for discussion in an environment where they will not be overheard or casually interrupted. The first communication attempts may be extremely difficult for the couple, and the nurse can warn both persons that they may be surprised and even hurt by their partner's interpretation of their behavior. The fact that they have not communicated or have misunderstood each other's actions will only underscore the essential place of improved communication in their sexual relationship.

Employing touching and physical closeness may also help bridge the gap created by poor communication. Some couples may have become so isolated from each other that even loving touching and basic physical contact are no longer a meaningful part of their daily lives. Reestablishing this important link can be an important part of improving overall communication.

Symptom Management
The area of symptom management offers the nurse multiple opportunities for successful intervention with patients. These interventions may be problem specific or handled in the form of anticipatory counseling to prevent the development of future problems. Three general areas that are applicable to arthritis patients are comfort strategies, positioning strategies, and alternatives to intercourse.

Comfort
Comfort is a critical area for patients with arthritis and one that clearly illustrates the importance of good communication. The fear of experiencing or inflicting pain can be a serious deterrent to satisfying sex for both partners. An early step in the communication process should be the establishment of a verbal or physical signal that can be used to alert the partner to the presence of serious pain. This allows the couple to pause, reposition, or simply lessen the intensity of the activity without having to abandon the sex act entirely. This sounds very simple, but it is crucial that this signal be given if pain occurs. The partner can then relax and enjoy the sex act without having to worry about whether verbal sounds of pleasure are instead indications of pain.

Other comfort strategies that are a part of the overall arthritis treatment regimen can also be employed to increase the patient's comfort during sexual activity. Spontaneity is only rarely an effective route to satisfying sex for arthritis patients. Basic planning can significantly increase the patient's comfort and pleasure.

Patients should consider planning sexual activity for the times of day when they are most comfortable and experiencing least fatigue. For many patients, this optimal time period is in the middle of the day rather than at night. Medication hours should also be evaluated and adjusted so that the patient is experiencing peak sustained pain relief during sexual activity. When strategies are sufficiently successful to allow participation in sexual activity, the act itself can contribute to the patient's comfort. The physical activity of sex stimulates the release of the body's own steroids and suppresses pain. In addition, sexual climax has been shown to produce an analgesic effect that may persist for several hours in some individuals and serves as an excellent reinforcer of natural sexuality.

The application of heat can also be used to increase the patient's comfort level during sexual activity. The use of heat may take the form of tub baths, showers, or warm packs and can be planned to involve the partner and become an integral part of sexual expression. Gentle massage can also be used to relax muscles and increase the flexibility of the joints. These techniques can become erotic exchanges when employed by a loving partner. Some couples find that the use of a water bed decreases the muscle fatigue of intercourse and frequently increases the degree of arousal.

All female patients can profit from incorporating isometric Kegel exercises into their daily exercise regimen. Since these exercises strengthen the pelvic musculature, they increase the ability of the vagina to grasp and squeeze the penis. This skill greatly increases the woman's ability to satisfy her partner when hip involvement negates vigorous pelvic thrusting.

Positioning

The attempt to find comfortable positions for sex is closely linked to the couple's ability to communicate successfully about sexual activity. When traditional sexual positions are either painful or physically impossible, the couple must be assisted to explore alternatives. For some couples, this type of exploration may challenge their accepted views of male/female sexual behavior, as well as their social mores about sex. But it is essential that this exploration be facilitated, as the issue of positioning can be very important. The traditional "missionary" position, with the woman on her back with her knees bent and legs spread wide and the man on top, is very likely to be extremely uncomfortable or impossible for women with hip or knee involvement or for men with arthritis affecting the knees, the joints of the arm, or the back.

More comfortable positions can be found if the couple is willing to experiment cautiously. Creative uses of pillows or furniture for lovemaking can significantly increase comfort and success. Since individual couples vary greatly in terms of physical size, relative weight, and disease involvement, it is not valuable to offer prescriptive advice to any couple about positioning. They will need to make the necessary evaluations themselves. In general, however, if the partner with arthritis is limited in movement, the position chosen should allow the other partner a moderate degree of freedom of movement. Again, the emphasis should be placed on the goal. Most couples can find a satisfactory and comfortable position for intercourse.

The following information about positioning is adapted from the Arthritis Foundation's pamphlet "Living and Loving" and offers specific positioning suggestions for persons with common disease restrictions (see Figure 4-1a–g).

Female Hip Involvement. The back-to-front position shown in Figure 4-1a is comfortable for many patients with hip involvement. With both partners lying on their side, minimal hip abduction capability is required for the male to enter from the rear. Pillows may be used to adjust angles and relieve pressure, but the position may not be possible if the woman cannot tolerate the weight on her shoulders or upper arms.

A kneeling position (Figure 4-1b), with the woman's upper body supported by furniture or pillows, is also quite successful when there is hip involvement. The man enters from the rear. This position again involves some pressure on the upper body, which may negate its use if the woman also has painful shoulder involvement.

A standing position (Figure 4-1c) may be less stressful for some couples. The woman positions herself comfortably over furniture of an appropriate height, using pillows as needed for cushioning. The man enters from the rear, putting minimal body weight on his partner.

Female Hip and Knee Involvement. A woman who has both hip and knee involvement or who cannot readily abduct her legs may wish to experiment with a back-lying position with support under the hips and thighs (Figure 4-1d). The male partner needs to support his own body weight on his hands and knees to reduce pressure.

The back-lying position pictured in Figure 4-1e may be attempted by women with severe disease and with hip contractures. In this position, the woman's knees are flexed and the man is positioned on his side, entering from the rear.

Male with Joint Involvement. The positions described for women with significant joint involvement can also frequently be comfortably used by men with arthritis, depending on the joints involved and the severity of the disease process. The kneeling, standing, and side-lying positions can often be comfortably employed.

A side-lying position with the partners facing each other (Figure 4-1f) may be useful if the man has significant back involvement. When

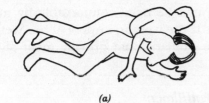

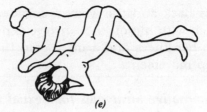

(a)

(e)

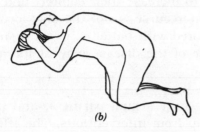

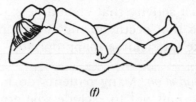

(b)

(f)

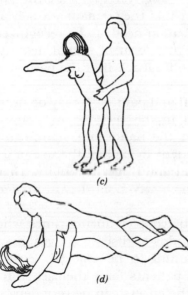

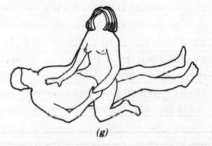

(c)

(g)

(d)

Figure 4–1. (a) Side-lying position; (b) kneeling position; (c) standing position; (d) back-lying position with hip and thigh support; (e) back-lying position; (f) side-lying position, partners facing; and (g) female astride position. (Adapted with permission from The Arthritis Foundation, *Arthritis—living and loving.* Atlanta: The Arthritis Foundation, 1982.)

this position is used, the woman assumes responsibility for providing most of the hip movement.

A female-dominant position (Figure 4-1g), with the man lying on his back and the woman astride, can be used comfortably by most men with hip or knee involvement if the woman supports her weight on her knees and arms. Again the woman must provide most of the hip movement.

Alternative Strategies for Sexual Fulfillment

Most of the preceding discussion has been focused on the strategies that may be employed by patients to increase their comfort and enjoyment during intercourse. But intercourse is not the only form of sexual activity that should be explored with patients. Certain situations that occur during the course of the disease may temporarily make intercourse inappropriate.

Masturbation. Many patients do not have sexual partners, and it is important not to exclude this group from interventions. The effects of their arthritis are just as devastating, yet they lack the support and validation from a loving partner that they remain sexually attractive. For these individuals, masturbation needs to be recognized and supported as a healthy and satisfying form of sexual activity that provides pleasure as well as positive feedback that the patient is still very much a sexual being.

If the patient's joints are very stiff and painful, it may be necessary to employ the methods addressed in the section on "Comfort" to prepare for pleasurable sex. When the hands are significantly involved, it may be useful for the patient to explore the use of a hand held vibrator to substitute for hand and finger flexibility. These devices need to be used with caution, however, as they are potentially irritating to delicate tissues.

Masturbation can also be used by couples during times when intercourse is not feasible. Exacerbations of disease activity may temporarily make intercourse too painful to be enjoyed, even when comfort strategies are employed. If patients force themselves to have intercourse during these periods, the effects can be very detrimental to the sexual relationship. Sexual pleasure, however, can still be given and received during these times through touching and mutual masturbation. The pleasure of giving sexual satisfaction to a partner can be extremely gratifying to the patient even when he or she is temporarily disinterested in the sex act itself. In this way, sexual activity remains an important aspect of the total expression of love and caring between the partners.

Oral sex. Oral sex is another obvious alternative to intercourse that is often not as physically demanding as intercourse. However, the practice may not have been a part of the patient's regular sexual experience and therefore needs to be introduced to the couple with sensitivity. The nurse's willingness to introduce the possibility of oral sex may help to foster its acceptability to couples who have never experimented with it. As with all forms of sexual activity, open communication between the partners is essential as they carefully explore and define the limits of their pleasure.

Abstinence. Specific portions of arthritis treatment protocols may also require the patient to explore alternative forms of sexual activity for limited periods of time. The patient with total joint replacement must refrain from intercourse for several weeks after surgery to prevent prosthesis dislocation. The temporary use of high dose steroids may increase the risk of pathologic fracture to the point where intercourse is contraindicated. The nurse needs to include these sexual issues in her teaching plan and introduce the idea of alternative patterns of sexuality for these times.

Birth Control

While the focus of the nurse's interventions is clearly on providing the information and encouragement necessary for patients to resume or improve their pattern of sexual activity, it would be remiss not to include counseling about birth control. Individuals with arthritis are confronted with so many changes and challenges that it is easy for them to lose sight of the realities of birth control and pregnancy. As always, the goal is to ensure that pregnancy, if it occurs, is a planned, conscious act and not merely an outcome of poor planning or oversight.

The woman with arthritis faces unique limitations in regard to birth control. The nature of her treatment protocol may negate the use of birth control pills. An intrauterine device remains an acceptable modality if her body tolerates it well. The use of a diaphragm, however, requires a fair degree of finger dexterity and hip flexibility for insertion. A tubal ligation is the easiest option if the woman does not wish to have additional children. Otherwise a woman must depend on her partner. A vasectomy will, of course, provide full protection, but the use of condoms is not very effective and probably should not be relied upon unless the woman is also capable of inserting a vaginal cream or foam. Decisions about birth control should be reached after full discussion between the partners.

The issue of sexuality for patients with arthritis is a challenging and important one for the nurse because it is an essential yet underserved area of patient care. It is relatively easy to put aside sexuality as a concern and delude ourselves that we are providing comprehensive care to our patients. But this is not an accurate perception. Sexuality is an integral part of our existence as men and women and an important component of adult relationships. Arthritis attacks a patient's sexuality in many ways as it creates changes in the patient's body image, self-esteem, role performance, and general physical functioning. Sexuality is an essential aspect of the activities of daily living. The nurse can be of significant help to the patient as she works to improve communication between the partners and to provide the couple with factual information and suggestions aimed at improving sexual functioning. But probably the most important nursing intervention involves communicating to the patient that continued sexual functioning is an appropriate concern and that the nurse is willing to serve as a resource in problem solving. Table 4-3 summarizes the basic interventions concerning sexuality in a care plan format.

Table 4–3   Care Plan Concerning Sexuality

Nursing Diagnosis	Patient Goal	Interventions
Altered patterns of sexuality related to altered body image and function secondary to arthritis.	Patient will regularly engage in sexual activity of his/her choosing and express satisfaction with sexual functioning. Patient and sexual partner will communicate openly concerning their sexual activities.	1. Complete sexual assessment, including: Normal pattern of sexual activity. Effect of arthritis on sexual activity and satisfaction. Patient's perceptions of and response to arthritis. Spouse's reaction to arthritis and its impact on sexuality. 2. Ensure privacy and reassure patient about confidentiality of data.

Table 4–3   Care Plan Concerning Sexuality (*Cont.*)

Nursing Diagnosis	Patient Goal	Interventions
		3. Assist patient and sexual partner to discuss their sexual relationship, including: Needs. Perceived problems. Establishing what is pleasurable and satisfying and what is not.
		4. Reinforce the importance of ongoing, frank communication about sex.
		5. Encourage partners to use touch and physical closeness to assist in bridging communication gaps.
Lack of knowledge related to specific techniques that can increase comfort with and satisfaction of the sexual relationship.	Patient will be able to state specific strategies that can increase comfort levels during sex. Patient and partner will incorporate comfort strategies into their patterns of sexual activity. Patient and partner will discuss alternative approaches to sexual activity and incorporate appropriate methods into their sexual routines.	1. Discuss with patient strategies that can increase the comfort level, including: Establishing a signal indicating the presence of serious pain. Planning sex for times of day when the patient is most comfortable and not fatigued. Modifying medication times to provide peak coverage during sexual activity. Experimenting with the use of heat or massage as part of the foreplay to intercourse.

continued

Table 4–3   Care Plan Concerning Sexuality (*Cont.*)

Nursing Diagnosis	Patient Goal	Interventions
		2. Teach female patients to incorporate Kegel exercises into their total exercise regimen.
		3 Provide patient with information about sexual positions that may increase comfort during intercourse.
		4. Initiate discussion with patient about alternative approaches to sexual activity that may be appropriate, including: Masturbation: alone, with partner, use of vibrators. Oral sex.
		5. Ensure that patient is using an effective method of birth control. Provide additional teaching as indicated.

CASE STUDIES

1. Meg Fisher is a 23-year-old white woman with rheumatoid arthritis. The disease was diagnosed shortly after her marriage and has not yet been adequately controlled by medication. Her husband is currently unemployed, and she is being seen in the arthritis clinic. As you review her general drug and exercise regimen, she suddenly bursts into tears. She states that over the last few weeks she has been experiencing severe pain in her right hip, which has made traditional intercourse impossible. Her husband is frightened and "turned off" by her pain. She had hoped that the physicians would recommend surgery to "fix" the problem, but they have informed her that the damage is not yet extensive enough to warrant surgery. She is desperate for help, stating that without sex she doesn't think her marriage will last much longer.

1. What kind of data should be gathered during this initial assessment?
2. How will you elicit this information from Meg? What kinds of questions will you ask?
3. What immediate interventions can you make with Meg to begin to deal with the problem?
4. What long-range goals and strategies might be appropriate?
5. Are there any community or professional resources that might be useful in this situation?

2. Bill Jones is a 43-year-old married man who was diagnosed as having rheumatoid arthritis 3 years ago. He has experienced several acute flare-ups during this period and has just been prescribed a regimen of gold injections, which will be administered and monitored by the community health nurse. You are meeting with Bill and his wife to attempt to establish an acceptable schedule for administration. Bill is a long-distance trucker and is often out of town. His job is taking a tremendous physical toll on him, but he feels that he has few other ways to match his current income with his skills. The Jones' have three boys aged 7, 11, and 12.

During your visit, Bill is called to the phone and Mrs. Jones blurts out her real concerns. She and her husband haven't had sex in months. Bill is constantly complaining of exhaustion, has a lot of hip and knee pain when he stops driving, and, in her view, gives all his extra time to the boys and their various scouting and sports activities. She feels that she is raising the boys alone and might as well not have a husband She doesn't know how much longer she can tolerate this situation.

1. What are the problems in this situation? Which of them are appropriate areas for nursing intervention?
2. What additional assessment data do you need to begin to formulate a plan of care? What questions will you ask to get the data you need?
3. What goals would be appropriate to establish at this time? What are the long-range goals?
4. Where will your interventions begin?
5. What resources might you use to intervene successfully in this situation?

PATIENT EDUCATION MATERIALS

Ayrault, E. W. (1981). *Sex, love and the physically handicapped.* Crossroad/Continuum Publishing Co., 575 Lexington Ave., New York, NY 10022.

Boggs, J. A. (1982). *Living and loving: Information about sex.* Arthritis Foundation, 1314 Spring St., NW, Atlanta, GA 30309.

Campling, J. (1981). *Images of ourselves: Women with disabilities talking.* Routledge & Kegan Paul, 9 Park St., Boston, MA 02108.

Duffy, Y. (1981). *All things are possible.* A. J. Garvin & Associates, Box 7525, Ann Arbor, MI 48107.

Parker, D. (1983). *Sex: Learning to love it again.* Boots Pharmaceuticals, Inc., Box 2686, Grand Central Station, New York, NY 10163.

Petrakis, P. E. (1979). *Arthritis and sex.* Rosalind Russell Arthritis Center, University of California—San Francisco, 1142 Fifth Ave., San Francisco, CA 94143.

Pitzele, S. K. (1985). *We are not alone: Learning to live with chronic illness.* Thompson & Co., 1313 5th St., SE, Suite 301, Minneapolis, MN 55414.

Task Force on Concerns of Physically Disabled Women. (1978). *Toward intimacy: Family-planning and sexuality concerns of physically disabled women,* 2nd ed. Human Sciences Press, 72 Fifth Ave., New York, NY 10011.

FILMSTRIP

Concept Media. (1978). *Disabling and deforming conditions: Impact on sexuality.* Concept Media, Box 19542, Irvine, CA 92714.

BIBLIOGRAPHY

Banwell, B. F., & Ziebell, B. (1985). Psychological and sexual health in rheumatic diseases. In W. N. Kelley et al. (eds.), *Textbook of rheumatology,* 2nd ed. (pp. 497–511). Philadelphia: W. B. Saunders.

Boggs, J. A. (1982). *Living and loving: Information about sex.* Atlanta: Arthritis Foundation.

Brassel, M. P. (1984). Sexuality. In G. K. Riggs and E. P. Gall (eds.), *Rheumatic diseases: Rehabilitation and management* (pp. 329–339). Boston: Butterworths.

Buckwalter, K. C., Wernimont, T., & Buckwalter, J. A. (1982). Musculoskeletal conditions and sexuality. *Sexuality and Disability.* 5(4), 195–207.

Conine, T. A., & Evans, J. H. (1982). Sexual reactivation of chronically ill and disabled adults. *Journal of Allied Health,* 11(4), 261–270.

Elst, P. (1984). Sexual problems in rheumatoid arthritis and ankylosing spondylitis. *Arthritis and Rheumatism,* 27(2), 217–220.

Ferguson, K., & Figley, B. (1979). Sexuality and rheumatic disease, a prospective study. *Sexuality and Disability,* 2(2), 130–138.

Figley, B. A., Ferguson, K. J., Bole, G. G., & Kay, D. R. (1980). A comprehensive approach to sexual health in rheumatic disease. *Topics in Clinical Nursing, 1*(4), 69–74.

Hesling, K. (1974). *Not made of stone.* Springfield, Ill.: Charles C. Thomas.

Hogan, R. (1985). Human sexuality: A nursing perspective. East Norwalk, CT: Appleton & Lange.

Johnson, W. R. (1975). *Sex education and counseling of special groups.* Springfield, Ill.: Charles C. Thomas.

Katz, W. A. (1986). Sexuality and arthritis. In W. A. Katz (Ed.), *Rheumatic diseases, diagnosis and management,* 2nd ed. (pp. 1011–1020). Philadelphia: J. B. Lippincott.

Malek, C. J., & Brower, S. A. (1984). Rheumatoid arthritis: How does it influence sexuality? *Rehabilitation Nursing, 9*(6), 26–28.

Mathon, P. G. (1983). Sexuality and arthritis: Living and loving with a chronic disease. *American Rehabilitation, 9,* 31–32.

Richards, J. S. (1980). Sex and arthritis. *Sexuality and Disability, 3*(2), 97–104.

Robinson, H. S. (1979). *You asked about rheumatoid arthritis.* Vancouver, B.C.: Douglas & McIntyre.

Robmault, I. P. (1978). *Sex, society and the disabled.* Hagerstown, Md.: Harper & Row.

Task Force on Concerns of Physically Disabled Women. (1978). *Toward intimacy,* 2nd ed. New York: Human Sciences Press.

Task Force on Concerns of Physically Disabled Women. (1978). *Within reach: Providing family planning services to physically disabled women,* 2nd ed. New York: Human Sciences Press.

Woods, N. F. (1984). *Human sexuality in health and illness,* 3rd ed. St. Louis: C. V. Mosby.

Yoshino, S., & Uchida, S. (1981). Sexual problems of women with rheumatoid arthritis. *Archives of Physical Medicine and Rehabilitation, 62*(3), 122–123.

PART 3

COMFORT ALTERATIONS

COMFORT ALTERATIONS

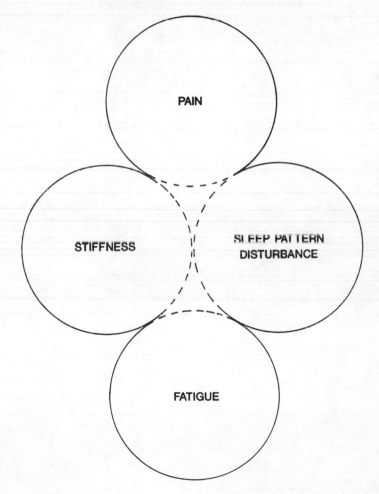

5

The Management of Arthritis Pain

Stephen T. Wegener
Cynthia Stabenow Kulp

Pain is a very common problem among patients with arthritis and is often the reason they seek medical treatment. The type of pain experienced can vary substantially with different forms of arthritis. Patients with rheumatoid arthritis may have intense pain during disease exacerbations but relatively little pain during periods of quiescence. Patients with generalized osteoarthritis, on the other hand, may experience low levels of chronic pain at all times, except when resting. Different types of pain require different types of management.

While it is clear that disease severity plays a major role in determining the intensity of the pain experienced, other factors may also influence both the pain and the patient's response. The experience of pain is influenced by other aspects of the rheumatic disease process as illustrated in the Pigg-Driscoll patient problems model (1985). Individuals in pain may experience sleep disturbances, which may lead to greater pain. High levels of fatigue and stiffness can also aggravate or intensify the pain. Pain can interfere with a patient's self-care abilities and mobility, as well as creating problems related to self-esteem. This chapter focuses on the role of pain in arthritis and on basic strategies for home management.

THE EXPERIENCE OF PAIN

Pain has been defined by the International Association for the Study of Pain as "an unpleasant sensory and emotional experience associated with actual or potential tissue damage or described in terms of such damage" (Mersky, 1979). While this description of pain is theoretically intriguing, it does not convey the personal suffering associated with a painful condition. Pain is unpleasant, but it is often much more than that. Pain is composed of multiple dimensions that can make individuals lose hope, cry, undergo serious operations, take dangerous medications, or, in a few cases, take their own lives. The simple adjective *unpleasant* cannot encompass the misery, desperation, and anguish that pain can produce. There are several important facts that are useful as a starting place for understanding pain.

Pain is not a discrete and quantifiable entity. Although the thresholds for pain perception and awareness appear to vary only minimally among individuals, the level of pain tolerance varies widely. One person with an inflamed joint may describe the pain as mild and relatively insignificant, while another may describe it as incapacitating and a reason for total inactivity. These differences in response may be due to sensory disease severity or to emotional or environmental factors that affect the reporting of pain. Previous experience with pain, as well as the person's cultural and family background, can affect pain tolerance. Individuals who have experienced other painful conditions may be able to place their arthritis pain in perspective and perceive it as less distressing. Past role models can also influence the person's response to pain. An arthritis patient who watched her mother "take to her bed" in response to arthritis pain may respond differently than one who observed family members continue to function in positive and adaptive ways.

The family and the support system can play a significant role in influencing a patient's response to disease. If the family reinforces activity limitation as an appropriate response to pain, this behavior is likely to become a hallmark of the patient's coping pattern. If, however, the family reinforces independence and adaptive self-care, the patient is less likely to fall victim to the negative outcomes of pain—anger, depression, inactivity, and withdrawal.

Finally, patients vary significantly in the degree of resourcefulness or helplessness that they bring to the pain experience. Some individuals rely totally on physicians and drugs, while others seek to control the pain experience through a variety of medical and self-management strategies. Community health nurses see the full range of responses to pain. Assisting patients to cope more effectively with their pain is one of the most important contributions nurses can make to arthritis home management.

Acute, Chronic, and Arthritis Pain

Pain in the broadest sense serves the function of informing us that something is wrong. Table 5-1 compares selected features of acute, chronic, and arthritis pain. Appropriate intervention strategies will be based on an understanding of the unique characteristics of each type of pain. Acute pain is the most common type encountered. The onset and the precipitating cause are usually specific, and there is a short time period during which the pain must be endured. Analgesics, rest, and limited activity are potential therapeutic components. Treatment usually controls the pain effectively and the person achieves relief, resuming previous activities.

Low back pain, recurrent headaches, and continuous pain due to benign medical problems are examples of chronic pain. In these situations, the cause of the pain may be unknown, the lesion uncertain, and the onset imprecise. Chronic pain typically has a long course (in

Table 5–1   Selected Features of Acute, Chronic, and Arthritis Pain

	Acute Pain	Chronic Pain	Arthritis Pain (Chronic and Intermittent)
Examples	Broken arm	Low back pain	Rheumatoid arthritis
Cause	Specific-onset and lesion	Variable-onset and lesion	Variable-onset and specific lesion
Course	Short	Long (6 months)	Long and recurring
Analgesics	Narcotic and nonnarcotic	Nonnarcotic if possible	Nonnarcotic if possible Temporary use of narcotics and steroids
Activity	Rest	Activity	Rest and activity
Exercise	Mild or restricted	Exercise as tolerated	Planned exercise
Usual outcome	Relief of pain	Continued pain	Continous, intermittent pain
Potential outcomes	Relief	Drug dependence Negative adaptation Behavioral changes	Learned helplessness Behavioral changes

excess of 6 months) and affects the individual's entire life. The biologic purpose of chronic pain is unclear, and it takes on a destructive quality. Narcotic analgesics are usually avoided with chronic pain, and patients are encouraged to remain as active as possible. Treatment is frequently unable to completely eliminate chronic pain, which can become an obsessive focus of the person's life. A destructive cycle involving the constant search for relief with little success is often repeated.

The pain associated with arthritis is complex. The pain of rheumatic diseases is often both chronic and intermittent. While pain is present continuously, it may vary in intensity from day to day. The pathology is specific and well defined, although the course of the disease is long, often with periods of exacerbation and relative remission. Medical management is complex, and the individual's response to the disease must be flexible. Rest and exercise must be planned and carefully balanced. The use of both narcotics and steroids is avoided if possible. The response to the treatment program is often unpredictable, and the individual is unlikely to get complete relief from pain.

Rheumatic Disease Pain Patterns

Persons with arthritis can demonstrate acute, chronic, and mixed forms of pain. Several of the major forms of rheumatic disease produce characteristic pain patterns (Dudley & Huskisson, 1972).

Osteoarthritis pain may be related to either cartilage damage or an accompanying inflammatory process. The characteristic pain associated with osteoarthritis is exacerbated by use and relieved by rest. Occasionally, osteoarthritis may involve an inflammatory process and result in a constant, deep, aching pain that is not relieved by rest.

Rheumatoid arthritis pain is extremely individual and reflects the complex nature of the disease process. Pain is associated with synovitis and inflammation of the joint. This pain is the result of pressure in the swollen joint capsule and may also be related to stiffness or impaired function. Typically, rheumatoid arthritis pain is described as aching, stabbing, and persistent. The daily pattern of the disease is such that the pain is often described as worse in the morning and may improve as the day progresses. It is not uncommon for individuals to report increased pain after activity, although it is unclear whether they are reporting increased pain or the impact of fatigue.

Gout pain is usually characterized by the sudden onset of localized, severe pain. This pain is related to the formation of uric acid crystals. Although it may be so excruciating that the slightest touch is unbearable, the course is relatively short, as pharmacologic interventions are effective in alleviating the condition.

Insufficient data have been collected on the pain patterns of systemic lupus erythematosus and ankylosing spondylitis, as these diseases are less common. In the case of juvenile rheumatoid arthritis, it has been observed that the disease appears to be less painful than the adult variety. This is surprising, given the devastating effects that the disease may have on joint function. The disease may actually be less painful or children may simply not be as effective in communicating their pain experience.

ASSESSMENT OF PAIN

Appropriate intervention for pain management depends on careful, ongoing pain assessment. The assessment of pain is one of the most difficult areas in nursing practice due to the subjective nature of pain. Blood pressure, temperature, and even the level of inflammation can be measured, but pain cannot. As McCaffery (1979) has written, "pain is whatever the patient says it is and is present whenever the patient says that it is" (p. 18). Nursing assessment of pain is therefore focused on assisting the patient to describe the nature and severity of the pain experience, the pain management strategies employed, and their relative effectiveness.

Pain information can be gathered in a variety of ways, including direct observations and reports from the patient and family. While sophisticated pain measurement tools are available, simple daily records are usually sufficient for community practice and maximize patient compliance. The community health nurse may maintain a record of semiobjective measures such as number of days in bed. It is often useful to have the patient keep a daily record of pain using a simple 1–10 numerical scale. The patient can record the pain status at intervals throughout the day, with 1 indicating no pain and 10 reflecting the severest pain. Family members can complete similar scales to document their perceptions. These data can be used to guide exercise and activity regimens and to monitor the patient's response to treatment.

Table 5-2 shows a weekly pain record that can be used to track a patient's pain, mood, and activity, as well as the pain management practices employed each day. The nurse can review these summaries during the home visit and plan modifications as needed.

The initial pain assessment process includes the gathering of other pertinent data, such as the location of the pain, its antecedents, the consequences of the pain for the patient's lifestyle and roles, and any pain treatments in current use. Careful interviewing is needed to establish what factors make the pain worse, what factors make it more bearable, and what the patient does in response to the pain. A better understanding of the individual's response to these events may help the nurse in planning the pain management program. It is also useful to obtain a list of treatments that have been tried in the past, including current medications and past analgesics, exercises, relaxation strategies, support groups, or other techniques

Table 5–2 Weekly Pain Assessment Tool

Each day, please pick a number between 0 and 10 to rate your pain level, mood, and activity restriction due to pain. Please also list what pain management strategies you used each day to help manage your pain.

Date	Pain Level	Mood Type	Activity Restriction	Pain Management Strategies Used
	0 is no pain 10 is pain as bad as it could be	0 is very good or happy; 10 is mood as bad or sad as it could be	0 is no restriction 10 is unable to do anything	
	_____highest _____lowest _____average	_____average	_____average	
	_____highest _____lowest _____average	_____average	_____average	
	_____highest _____lowest _____average	_____average	_____average	
	_____highest _____lowest _____average	_____average	_____average	
	_____highest _____lowest _____average	_____average	_____average	

that have been or are being used. An example of a comprehensive pain assessment questionnaire can be found in Table 5-3.

Table 5–3   Pain Assessment Inventory—Nurse Scale (Pains)

Date _____   Clinician _____
Patient Name _____   Location _____
Diagnosis _____   Patient Number _____

1. PAIN HISTORY
   A. When did this pain begin?   Year _____   Month _____
   B. Did this pain begin?   Gradually _____   Suddenly _____

2. Please choose a number between 0 and 100 where 0 is "no pain" and 100 is the "worst possible pain" to describe how strong your pain is.
   A. _____ Good days   A. _____ Average this month
   B. _____ Bad days   B. _____ Average this past week
                              C. _____ Today
                              D. _____ Worst pain you ever had
                                 What was it: _____

3. How much does it bother you?
   Now   0 1 2 3 4 5 6 7 8 9 10
              very little   very much
   Usually   0 1 2 3 4 5 6 7 8 9 10

4. PAIN PATTERN
   A. Do you have the pain immediately on waking? Yes _____ No _____
      If no, when does the pain begin? _____
   B. Does the pain change during the day? Yes _____ No _____
      If yes, what part of the day is the pain worse? _____
      What part of the day is the pain better? _____
   C. How long does your morning stiffness, if any, last? _____ hours

5. Rate yourself on each of the following items by placing a check mark in the block which best corresponds to your rating:
   A. How often do you experience pain from your arthritis?

1	2	3	4	5
Never	Seldom	Sometimes	Often	Constantly
____	____	____	____	____

   B. When is your pain the worst?

1	2	3	4	5
Lying down	Sitting	Standing	Walking	Bending/twisting
____	____	____	____	____

   C. How often are you confined to bed because of pain?

1	2	3	4	5
Never	Seldom	Sometimes	Often	Constantly
____	____	____	____	____

Table 5–3   Pain Assessment Inventory—Nurse Scale (Pains) (*Cont.*)

6. TREATMENT

   Please list all the treatments you have had and are currently having for your pain. Include operations, medications, physiotherapy and psychological treatments.

Name and Type of Treatment	Date Started	Type of Treatments and Number of Treatments (i.e., Once a Week/Every Day)	Effect	
			Helped	Did Not Help

7. PAIN MODIFIERS

   For each of the following, please mark with a + if it increases the pain; please mark with a − if it decreases the pain; please mark with a 0 if it has no effect on on your pain.

   ( ) splints   ( ) lying down   ( ) vigorous exercise
   ( ) cold   ( ) massage   ( ) walking
   ( ) sleep   ( ) mild exercise   ( ) weather
   ( ) braces   ( ) sitting   ( ) work
   ( ) heat   ( ) standing   ( ) others _____
   ( ) housework   ( ) relaxation   _____
   ( ) loud noises   ( ) season   _____

8. What activities bring on the pain, or make it worse? _____
   _____
   _____

9. Does rest decrease your pain? Yes _____ No _____ How many hours do you rest each day? _____

10. If I were there when you were in pain, what would I see and hear? How do people around you know when you are in pain? _____
    _____
    _____

continued

Table 5–3 Pain Assessment Inventory—Nurse Scale (Pains) *(Cont.)*

11. If I were there when you were in pain, how likely is it that I would know that you were having pain?

1	2	3	4	5
Never	Seldom	Sometimes	Often	Always
___	___	___	___	___

12. PAIN PROBLEMS

    During the past month, how much did pain interfere with the following activities? Circle the number for each of the questions that best describes your situation.

1	2	3	4	5
Not at all	A little bit	Moderately	Quite a bit	Extremely
___	___	___	___	___

Going to work	1	2	3	4	5
Performing household chores	1	2	3	4	5
Yard work or shopping	1	2	3	4	5
Socializing with friends	1	2	3	4	5
Recreation and hobbies	1	2	3	4	5
Having sexual relations	1	2	3	4	5
Physical exercise	1	2	3	4	5

13. When you are in pain, how often does your husband/wife/other family support and encourage you?

1	2	3	4	5
Never	Seldom	Sometimes	Often	Always
___	___	___	___	___

14. When you are in pain, how often does your husband/wife/other family ignore you or become angry?

1	2	3	4	5
Never	Seldom	Sometimes	Often	Always
___	___	___	___	___

15. Was any member of your family disabled from a pain or arthritis problem?

    Yes ( )   No ( )

    If yes, state relationship _____

    His/her problem _____

16. Anything else you want to say about your arthritis pain/stiffness

    _____
    _____
    _____

PAIN MANAGEMENT STRATEGIES

Self-Help Strategies in the Home

When a patient with arthritis is suffering from painful joints or morning stiffness, the patient and the family use any remedy available in the home to bring relief. An examination of the medicine cabinet may produce aspirin or some other pain medication. A "rub" may be applied to the painful area. A heating pad, electric blanket, or hot water bottle may be used to provide temporary relief. The strategies for pain management, though many and varied, are rarely applied with any organized, consistent problem-solving approach designed to provide pain relief. After completing a careful pain assessment, the nurse can assist the patient and family to devise a coordinated, effective pain management program for safe use in the home.

Patient Education

The first step in the implementation of any treatment plan involves patient and family education concerning the nature of the condition and how the treatment program will work. For arthritis pain management, this means educating patients about the nature of their pain and about what can be done in treatment. The unique challenges of arthritis pain need to be explained. The nurse acknowledges the reality of the pain and helps patients to understand that it will be influenced by many physical, social, and environmental factors. She emphasizes that there are many physical, mental, and pharmacologic strategies that can be used to help manage the arthritis pain. There is hope. Table 5-4 presents a patient information sheet on pain management that reviews various aspects of pain management that may be useful to include in the patient education process.

Table 5—4   Patient Information on Pain Management

What pain means and how it is experienced varies from person to person. It is not always possible to either pinpoint the exact cause of pain or, unfortunately, relieve it entirely. However, it is possible to learn to manage pain through the use of a wide variety of measures. What works for one person may not work for the next. What works at one time may not work at another time. What is important to remember is that there is something that can be done about pain.

continued

Table 5–4 Patient Information on Pain Management (*Cont.*)

Pain is not all bad. Pain is nature's signal that something is wrong. Pain sends one to see a doctor in the first place. Pain tells one to slow down, protect, or not to use a part. Some people do not have pain or do not seem to feel pain easily. They have no signal and are apt to injure and cause damage to themselves. They, too, have a problem, but of a different sort.

Pain is a result of the disease process either directly or indirectly. It is important that the patient (and family) understand pain so that the ways in which it can be managed make sense. Pain can be caused directly by the release of a substance (histamine) that irritates the nerve endings. This change happens as a part of the inflammatory process. Inflammation also causes a greater release of fluid into the tissues. This process is recognizable as swelling. Sometimes it is not possible to control inflammation completely, or a degenerative process occurs leading to a malalignment of the joint or a wearing away of the cartilage at the ends of the bones. This results in a mechanical problem and pain. The muscles, tendons, or ligaments can be affected. Spasm can also result in pain.

There are many ways of managing pain. Exactly why these methods work is not always known; they may work in a combination of ways. The following is a list of measures that can help manage pain.

Physical measures
  Application of heat or cold
  Counterirritants such as liniments or creams; transcutaneous electrical nerve
    stimulantion devices
  Massage (light stroking)
  Positioning
Mental measures
  Relaxation techniques
  Distraction
  Imagery
Pharmacologic measures
  Analgesics
  Antidepressants
  Muscle relaxants

Often a person must try a variety of real life measures to find what works best. Experiment—what is there to lose? A combination of measures may be helpful.

Source: Pigg, J.S., Driscoll, P.W., & Caniff, R. *Rheumatology Nursing*. Copyright © 1985 John Wiley & Sons, Inc. Reprinted by permission of John Wiley & Sons, Inc.

The education process helps to convince patients that the nurse takes their pain seriously and is committed to developing an effective treatment plan. It also conveys the message that the treatment plan will be a partnership in which the patient must play a central role. Developing a personal pain plan can be an effective strategy for involving the patient in responsibility for pain management. When arthritis pain becomes severe, it can be difficult for patients to develop appropriate management strategies. Planning in *advance* how the patient will cope can be very effective. The personal pain plan shown in Table 5-5 suggests activities that the patient will do each day to prevent the pain from getting out of control. The plan includes activities chosen by the patient in conjunction with the nurse and other members of the health care team. It provides for both self-help and medical interventions and establishes a loose contract on how the patient will respond to pain. This chapter discusses a variety of methods that may be considered for inclusion in the personal pain plan.

Table 5-5   Personal Pain Plan

To help me manage my arthritis pain better, I will do the following activities:

1. Medications to help my pain are: I take the medications at these times:

_____   _____

_____   _____

_____   _____

_____   _____

2. Heat/cold/massage can help my pain.
   What I will do: When I will do it:

_____   _____

_____   _____

3. Rest is important in managing my pain.
   I will rest:
   Whole body rest   Time _____
   Specific joint rest   Time _____
   (_____) Fill in joint

4. Being calm and relaxed helps the pain. My way to practice relaxation is: _____. I will practice _____ times each day.

5. Keeping my mind off the pain is important. When in pain I will think about: (List some pleasant thoughts or memories.)

_____   _____

_____   _____

continued

Table 5–5   Personal Pain Plan (*Cont.*)

6. I need to keep my life focused on healthy habits such as making sure that I eat lots of fresh fruit and vegetables. One new healthy habit I'm going to practice is: _____

7. Exercise is important in controlling pain. My exercise plan is: _____

_____

8. The ideas for pain control I am going to ask my doctor about are: _____

_____

Fill out this Personal Pain Plan and put it somewhere you will see it—the refrigerator door or dresser mirror.

Source: Stephen Wegener, Ph.D., 1986. All rights reserved.

Physical Modalities

Thermal (Heat) Strategies. Many forms of heat are available over the counter for home use. Patients with long-standing arthritis may have used various forms of heat and have strong ideas about which type or combination is best for them. Table 5-6 lists common forms of heat that can safely and comfortably be used in the home. The nurse can encourage patients to experiment with new or alternative approaches and assist them to evaluate their effectiveness appropriately.

Whenever a heat modality is used in the home, certain guidelines should be followed to ensure safety. An application of heat should not exceed 15–20 minutes at a time. Patients who use heat for longer periods risk burning their skin. The nurse should encourage the patient to use heat at intervals throughout the day rather than for one prolonged period. Thermal strategies work by increasing blood flow to the affected part and altering the threshold of pain perception. Prolonged heat application neither adds to nor extends the inhibition of pain impulses. Most home methods use moist heat rather than dry heat, since it penetrates more deeply yet does not raise the temperature as high and is less likely to cause burning. Special care must be employed to ensure safety when dry heat is used.

Some heat modalities for home use are heavy or awkward for patients with hand deformities (e.g., hot water bottles, hot packs). The application of a heavy heat modality may actually increase the patient's pain due to the weight. The nurse can teach the patient to use alternative strategies that produce the same relief without the added weight and stress.

Table 5–6 Examples of Common Heat Modalities

Modality	Considerations
1. Warm shower or tub bath	Often overlooked but an economical comfort modality Provides relaxation in addition to warmth for pain management Shower bench and grab bars are necessary for patient safety
2. Hot water bottle	Readily available and economical for home use May be heavy and awkward to apply More than one may be needed for multiple joint involvement
3. Heating pad	Readily available and economical for home use Dry or moist heat options in the same heating pad are preferable Limited coverage for painful body areas
4. Dampened towel placed in microwave oven for 15–30 seconds	Readily available and economical heat modality if microwave is available Can provide optimal heat to many joints Contours to curved body surfaces
5. Hot pack	Assistance from family members may be needed to prepare and apply this modality Frequent skin checks and multiple layers of towels may be necessary to avoid burns
6. Paraffin dip (for hands or feet) (see Table 5-7 for preparation of paraffin at home)	Readily available and economical heat modality Assistance from family members may be needed to prepare paraffin bath
7. Contrast bath (for hands or feet) (see Table 5-8 for proper sequence and water temperature	Readily available and economical heat modality Can increase circulation in hands and feet

Heat modalities should never be combined. The use of an ointment or linament in conjunction with a heating pad or hot pack can significantly increase the patient's chance of burning the skin. The nurse needs to assess the patient's home use of heat in depth and provide both written and oral instructions about correct and safe usage. Supervised practice is always desirable and may be essential for those with limited literacy.

Many elderly patients with arthritis have coexistent medical problems resulting in poor peripheral circulation *and* decreased sensation. The nurse needs to assess the patient's skin integrity before suggesting a home program that will use heat modalities. She also needs to emphasize the safety precautions that must be employed whenever heat is used. Serious burns are a real possibility.

Sometimes patients feel that if a little is good, more is better. This applies to both the intensity and the duration of heat. The nurse needs to monitor initial applications of heat and reinforce her teaching as needed until the patient and family use the method with confidence and safety.

As shown in Table 5-6, there are many heat modalities available for home use. The nurse and patient need to determine which modalities are most effective. The nurse should consult with the physician and physical therapist as needed concerning any specific precautions that patients need to follow in their use of heat. See Tables 5-7 and 5-8 for patient information sheets on the use of paraffin baths and contrast baths.

Cold Strategies. Although cold is not usually thought of as a comfort strategy, it can provide dramatic pain relief for some patients. It is particularly effective for the acute pain of hot, inflamed joints. The nurse can encourage patients to experiment with its use. Cold appears to work by slowing or blocking the transmission of pain impulses to the brain.

In the home, cold is usually delivered by cold or slush pack or by means of an ice massage. Except for intermittent ice massage, ice should never be placed directly against the skin. A cloth barrier should always be in place. As a general rule, ice should not be used for more than 10–15 minutes at a time, although it may be reapplied at frequent intervals. Longer use may produce frostbite, and any cold pack should be removed once the numbing effect occurs. The patient should use light-weight cold packs to avoid pressure damage and probably should not be encouraged to use ice at all if circulatory problems exist.

Table 5–7   Patient Information Sheet: Paraffin Bath

Equipment

1 double boiler
6 pounds of canning paraffin
1/2 cup mineral oil
1 thermometer, with scale marking about 130°F
1 plastic bag per hand or plastic food wrap
1 heavy turkish towel per hand

Preparation of Wax

1. Fill lower part of double boiler with water and heat.
2. Cut the 6 pounds of paraffin into pieces and place in upper part of double boiler.
3. When paraffin is about melted, add the 1/2 cup of mineral oil and stir.
4. Because paraffin is flammable, remove pan from stove and let the bath cool.
5. Use only when the temperature is 120–130°F.
   Caution: When checking the temperature, be certain thermometer is not touching the bottom of the pan.

Preparation of Patient

1. Inspect the hand to be treated for the condition of the skin. Paraffin should not be applied over open cuts or sores.
2. Cleanse the hand thoroughly with soap and water.

Treatment

1. Holding the hand in a comfortable position, immerse it in the paraffin, being careful not to touch the bottom of the pan. Then remove and allow the paraffin to harden.
   Caution: Do not move the fingers or wrist so as to crack the paraffin during the dipping procedure.
2. Repeat the dipping 5 to 10 times until the glove is about 1/4 inch thick.
3. Optional: After glove forms, immerse hand and wrist in paraffin for 20 minutes.
4. Remove from bath and place hand in a plastic wrap.
5. Then wrap in a heavy turkish towel.
6. Leave the glove on the hand for 20 minutes.

Removal of Wax

1. Run forefinger down the inside of the glove and peel wax off.
2. Empty perspiration from the glove.
3. Return glove to pan for reuse.

Source: Reprinted with permission from the Midwest Arthritis Treatment Center, Columbia Hospital, Milwaukee, WI.

Table 5–8 Patient Information Sheet: Contrast Baths

Use two bins of water, one cool (approximately 59°F) and one warm (approximately 104°F). Total treatment time is 30 minutes. Start and finish treatment in warm water. Immerse hands in warm water for specified time, then in the cool water. Alternate for a total of 30 minutes.

Warm water	10 min
Cool water	1 min
Warm water	3-4 min
Cool water	1 min
Warm water	4 min
Cool water	1 min
Warm water	4 min
Cool water	1 min
Warm water	4 min

Source: Reprinted with permission from the Midwest Arthritis Treatment Center. Columbia Hospital, Milwaukee, WI.

CONTRAST BATHS. This cold modality lends itself well to home use because it is convenient and involves minimal cost. Many arthritis patients are aware of the benefits of warm water soaks, even during dish washing, for increasing flexibility when hands are painful. Combining the use of warm water with cold water, however, is often a novel idea for patients, and the cold water immersion may require some coaxing. This thermal modality is often beneficial for patients with rheumatoid arthritis who experience significant morning stiffness. It may also benefit patients with inflammatory osteoarthritis of the hands. Contrast baths can be effectively combined with ROM exercises in the water or with resistive exercises such as squeezing a sponge or nerf ball under water.

Massage. Scientific evidence to support or document the role of massage in pain management is lacking, but a great deal of subjective evidence points to the benefits of massage when patients are in pain. It is possible that cutaneous stimulation may help to alter the pain cycle through the release of body endorphins (endogenous opiates) or through the stimulation of certain nerve fibers that help to block pain transmission. Nurses have used touch and massage at the bedside for many years.

   Massage may be employed as a valuable pain treatment modality in the home. Patients automatically rub painful body parts in an attempt to reduce pain, increase circulation, or even "warm up" the affected part. A loving family member can often calm a patient experiencing pain with gentle massage, especially when it is combined with another modality or medication. Light, gentle massage can usually be safely used in the home.

Positioning. Nurses and therapists often see the flexion contractures that can result from the improper use of positioning in the home. Patients accommodate painful joints by propping pillows behind the head, knees, and elbows. While this positioning technique is an effective pain relief strategy, it can have disastrous results in the form of joint contractures when the pain subsides.

The nurse should assess the patient's preferred sleeping and sitting postures at home and examine the bed or chair being used. Sometimes patients sleep in a chair at night because it is more comfortable. Family members may need instruction and education regarding correct positioning to avoid flexion contractures in painful joints. A neutral position with the joints in extension is the goal. Bed mattresses should be very firm or bed boards should be in place. One small, flat pillow under the head is all that should be used, and pillows should never be placed under painful knees. The immobilization of painful joints controls pain by limiting movement. The use of local splints may be useful, allowing the part to rest while ensuring that the joint is maintained in a position of function. The use of splints is discussed in Chapter 3, along with the role that occupational therapists can play in assisting the nurse to solve a positioning problem in the home.

It is important to be realistic in the management of the home program. Getting a good night's sleep is a priority for most arthritis patients. If the patient needs to assume a flexed posture for sleep in order to be comfortable, the nurse can suggest a positioning program of splints or lying prone at intervals during the day to combat the effects of flexed knees, hips, or elbows from a night of sleep. Figure 5-1 illustrates a beneficial resting or sleeping posture that should be encouraged if the patient can tolerate it.

Psychologic Modalities

Relaxation. Some persons with arthritis find that relaxation training is useful in managing their pain. Pain is often accompanied by muscle tension, shallow breathing, and blood flow restriction, as well as by the emotions of anxiety and tension. Many patients believe that

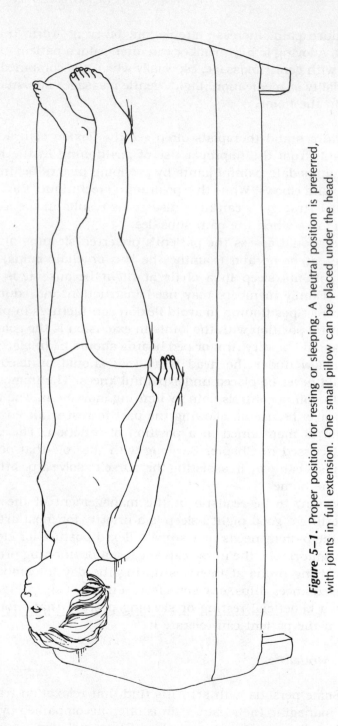

Figure 5–1. Proper position for resting or sleeping. A neutral position is preferred, with joints in full extension. One small pillow can be placed under the head.

stress makes their arthritis worse, and there are scientific observations to suggest that stressful events may be associated with the perception of greater pain (Sternbach, 1978).

While the scientific literature is not extensive, there are data to support the idea that relaxation lessens the perception of pain in persons with arthritis (Bradley et. al., 1984; Wegener, 1986). Exactly how relaxation is effective in alleviating arthritis pain is not known. It has been postulated that the mechanism may involve release of endorphins, distraction of attention from the pain, reduction of muscle tension, or reduction of anxiety. While the research is ongoing, relaxation continues to be a useful pain management strategy.

Several methods can be used to develop the relaxation response. These include progressive muscle relaxation, deep breathing, autogenic training, self-hypnosis, imagery, biofeedback, meditation and even prayer.

Deep breathing is the basis for many relaxation techniques and is often a useful place to begin when teaching relaxation training. There is no one best way to relax. It may be necessary to try different methods until one is found that is most effective and acceptable to the patient. Table 5-9 provides an outline for basic deep breathing exercise.

Table 5–9   Guidelines for Deep Breathing

This exercise can be practiced in a variety of positions, but lying down on a bed or sitting in a supportive chair is recommended. This exercise can be learned in a few minutes, but regular practice is necessary to maximize the benefits. If you are working with someone, explain the advantages of deep breathing, namely, increased blood oxygenation, decreased muscle tension, improved circulation to the periphery, and attention directed away from the pain.

1. Place one hand on the abdomen and one hand on your chest.
2. Inhale slowly and deeply through your nose. Notice which hand rises first. (Most people find that the chest hand rises first, indicating shallow, ineffective, constricted breathing.)
3. Again place one hand on the chest and one on the abdomen. Inhale slowly through the nose, trying to cause the hand on the abdomen to rise first. This should be done naturally by breathing, not by actively distending the muscles. When it is done correctly, the abdomen rises first, followed by a slight chest rise. In some cases, the increase in oxygen may make the person dizzy or upset. These persons should be cautioned to proceed slowly, not forcing the breathing but supporting a slow, natural process.

Table 5–9   Guidelines for Deep Breathing (*Cont.*)

4. Once abdominal breathing is established, make sure that breathing is nice and slow. This can be facilitated by breathing in through the nose, pausing, and exhaling slowly through the mouth. Focus on the sound and feeling of breathing as you become more and more relaxed.
5. Next, make sure that the breathing is smooth. Your breathing should be similar to the gentle waves of the ocean; gently allow air to flow in and out without long pauses.
6. Practice three times per day. Each practice session should last for about 5 minutes. Some people find it helpful to count breaths. If you do this, practice until you count to 100. Each time you exhale, say to yourself words like *relax, calm, or warm.*

TYPES OF RELAXATION STRATEGIES

Progressive muscle relaxation (PMR) usually involves alternately tensing and releasing specific muscle groups in a progressive order. This helps the person learn the difference between tension and relaxation. PMR is commonly used as part of the training for prepared childbirth and is a technique familiar to nurses. A number of the readings in the bibliography at the end of this chapter provide specific instructions for detailed PMR training. PMR can place excessive stress on inflamed joints, and patients who use it should be cautioned not to strain their joints. A more passive method such as autogenic training or imagery may be more helpful.

AUTOGENIC TRAINING INVOLVES

Inducing a relaxed state by repeating phrases that suggest relaxation in various parts of the body. Specific instructions for this procedure are included in Table 5-10. This may be a helpful exercise, as it does not stress joints and may be focused on particular parts of the body.

IMAGERY

Involves the development of specific images in the mind to counteract or block pain. A relaxing scene is envisioned—a beach, meadow, or country road—and is focused in the mind's eye. It is important that the pleasant image be completely pictured. The individual should try to be aware of the details of the sights, sounds, textures, and smells, making the scene as real as possible. In an alternative approach, the image can be used to alleviate the pain in a symbolic way. For example, imagery can be useful when the person has hot, inflamed joints. The person might picture the pain as a setting sun—hot, red, and bright. As the person visualizes the sun slowly setting, the pain is felt

Table 5–10   Guidelines for Atuogenic Training

Instructions: Choose a quiet room where you won't be disturbed. Have the room at a comfortable temperature and wear loose clothing. Either sit in an armchair with your head, back, and arms supported or lie down with your head supported and arms resting comfortably at your sides. Begin by practicing 2 minutes of deep breathing exercises to set the stage for training.

It takes seven weeks to develop the response fully. Each week the program teaches a new skill.

Week 1

Repeat the following phrases for 5 minutes three times per day. Each phrase is repeated four times, and then the whole sequence is repeated. Each time you say a phrase, say it slowly and then pause for about 3 seconds.

>My right arm is heavy.
>My left arm is heavy.
>Both of my arms are heavy.

Week 2

Repeat the following for 5 minutes three times per day.

>My right arm is heavy.
>My left arm is heavy
>Both of my arms are heavy.
>My right leg is heavy.
>My left leg is heavy.
>Both of my legs are heavy.
>My arms and legs are
>heavy.

Week 3

Repeat the following for 8 minutes three times per day.

>My right arm is heavy.
>My arms and legs are
>heavy.
>My right arm is warm.
>My left arm is warm.
>Both of my arms are warm.

Week 4

Repeat the following for 10 minutes two times per day.

>My right arm is heavy.
>My arms and legs are heavy.

continued

Table 5–10   Guidelines for Atuogenic Training (*Cont.*)

My right arm is warm.
My left arm is warm.
My right leg is warm.
My left leg is warm.
Both of my legs are warm.
My arms and legs are warm.

Week 5

Repeat the following for 15 minutes two times per day.
My right arm is heavy.
My arms and legs heavy.
Both of my legs are warm.
My arms and legs are warm.
My arms and legs are heavy and warm.

Week 6

Repeat the following for 15 minutes two times per day.
My right arm is heavy.
My arms and legs are heavy.
My arms and legs are warm.
My arms and legs are heavy and warm.

Note: If you have trouble experiencing warmth using verbal phrases, try visual images. For example, imagine your arm in the sun or lying on a warm heating pad. Imagine your hand submerged in warm water or standing in a shower. When you are ready to stop the practice, say to yourself "When I open my eyes I will feel refreshed, relaxed, and alert." Then open your eyes, take a few breaths, and stretch your arms and legs. Make sure that you are in control of your muscles when you stand up.

Remember, it will take some time to get results. Enjoy the practice time. It is your time; think of nothing else. It is time to take care of yourself.

to diminish with it. The individual can visualize the sun setting again and again until he or she feels cool and relaxed.

Self-hypnosis is deep relaxation created by focusing attention completely on one thought or experience. Usually professional help is necessary to learn this skill. The ability to use self-hypnosis varies from person to person, and it may take some time to acquire the skill.

MEDITATION

Involves creating a relaxed state by concentrating on one thought, phrase, or image in a repetitive fashion. A number of meditation techniques are discussed in the bibliography at the end of this chapter. In some ways, prayer can be seen as a type of meditation relaxation, as the individual concentrates on one particular subject and often repeats a well-known prayer over and over. Often this prayerful state is accompanied by slow, regular breathing and the other physical forms of relaxation. It also focuses attention away from the pain.

Other relaxation training techniques, such as biofeedback and hypnosis, usually require professional expertise and are not applicable as basic self-help home strategies. These approaches and their applications are discussed in more detail later in the chapter.

Table 5-11 outlines some basic principles for relaxation training. In the beginning, it may be useful to practice with the patient. If the nurse is not comfortable with this technique, it is unlikely that she

Table 5–11   Guidelines for Relaxation Training

1. *Pick a quiet time and place.* A relaxation session will require at least 10 minutes that are not interrupted by noise from the television, radio, or other people. Soft instrumental music or the hum of an air conditioner can be used to muffle other noises.

2. *Sit or lie in a comfortable position with your head supported and eyes closed.* Remove eyeglasses; loosen constrictive clothing, ties, and splints.

3. *Begin with deep breathing exercises.* Deep breathing is the basis for other relaxation approaches and sets the stage for other strategies.

4. *Remain focused on breathing and relaxation.* If other thoughts come to mind, try to let these thoughts drift through like clouds, telling yourself, "I will think about that later."

5. *Don't worry about getting "relaxed."* Relaxation will come with practice. If nothing else, the rest is beneficial.

6. *Practice for 10–15 minutes two times per day until the relaxation response is firmly established.* Do not practice right after a meal. Don't worry if you fall asleep, but try to stay awake the next time. Once it is established, the relaxation response can be used whenever it is needed to escape from pain or relax in the face of stressful events.

will be successful in helping others. Some patients find it easier to use taped relaxation instructions. The nurse can prepare a tape for their use or patients can use commercially available tapes.

Common barriers to successful relaxation training include not taking sufficient time to practice, not believing that it will help, and feeling embarrassed during practice. Some patients are skeptical of these nonpharmaceutical techniques, as they are not tangible or familiar. Education concerning the purpose of relaxation training and practicing the relaxation exercise with the patient are critical strategies for overcoming these problems. Other patients may need help in structuring practice time. When working out an activity or pacing the schedule with the patient, the nurse can build in relaxation time. Patients may need to confront limitations in insight if they continually put their needs last. Strengthening their self-esteem and encouraging them to set aside time for themselves are critical. It is possible that relaxation may not be helpful in controlling their arthritis pain; however, the improved self-esteem that comes from practicing self-care is always beneficial.

Cognitive Interventions. How persons with arthritis conceptualize and think about their pain influences how they experience the pain. Research indicates that certain cognitive strategies may be useful in modifying the pain people experience (Turk, Meichenbaum, & Genest, 1983). These strategies fall into three groups—attention diversion, refocusing, and pain inoculation training. These strategies may be particularly helpful when the person needs to undergo an acute procedure such as intra-articular injection, fluid removal, or biopsy. They may also be useful when the person is experiencing a temporary increase in arthritis pain, either during a disease flare up or when joint pain increases secondary to overuse.

Some patients practice these techniques spontaneously. Others must be taught their use. Like other techniques, these skills must be practiced to be effective. Cognitive approaches may be viewed with skepticism, and patients must be convinced that they are able to redirect their attention to help control their environment. Distraction is real. We all fail to hear ringing telephones or verbal calls for attention when we are engrossed in activities such as reading or watching television. These techniques can be powerful tools, and yet they can be taught in the home. Table 5-12 provides guidelines similar to those developed by McCaffery (1979) and are useful in teaching any cognitive intervention strategy.

Table 5–12 Guidelines for Teaching Cognitive Strategies

1. *Assess what diversion strategies the person is using, how often they are being used, in what context, and how successful they are in modifying the pain.* In order to use these techniques, the patient must be able to concentrate and follow directions. These abilities should be assessed informally.

2. *Explain the rationale to the patient.* Describe the different approaches that are available and suggest one which you think may be initially helpful.

3. *Let the patient choose the strategy to use and decide when to use it.* This will increase the investment in the technique and improve the patient's sense of control over the disease.

4. *Try to teach and practice the strategy during periods of minimal or mild pain.* It is difficult to learn these techniques while in severe pain. Until the skill is well established, attempting its use to modify severe pain will result in discouragement.

5. *Use a relaxation technique such as deep breathing before the training.* This will enhance learning and aid in pain modification.

6. *Practice the strategy with the client.* Mere instruction is not sufficient; supervised practice is required.

7. *Explore the patient's concerns about using the strategy. Address these concerns with education if necessary.* Often the best way to deal with them is to practice the technique with the patient and talk about the experience afterward.

8. *Have the patient practice daily.* Ideally, the individual should practice two to three times per day, but at least once per day is necessary. Practice sessions need not be long; 10–15 minutes is often sufficient.

9. *Follow up during subsequent visits.* Your reinforcement of the practice and use of these strategies is critical. The community health nurse's attention is a powerful reinforcer.

ATTENTION DIVERSION

Where one's attention is focused can either amplify or reduce the perception of pain. Patients who withdraw from other activities and focus their attention on their pain frequently exacerbate its intensity. Others are able to reduce the impact of pain by focusing on other internal or external events.

IMAGERY

In addition to its use as a relaxation technique, imagery may be used as an attention diversion strategy. Persons may focus on and describe to themselves a particular book, movie, or scene that is very involving. Initially it may be useful to have the person describe the scene aloud while creating a mental picture of the scene. The person should be encouraged to involve as many senses as possible in order to intensify the experience. The goal here is not to eliminate pain but to move it to the background and let something else become the focus of attention. Other useful images may be a pleasant fantasy, a childhood memory, or a special comfortable place. The image can be changed as necessary to keep the person involved.

REFOCUSING

Pain may be diminished by refocusing attention away from the pain to something outside of oneself. Engaging in activities such as reading, watching television, or talking to others are all activities that distract attention from pain. This strategy is often used spontaneously to help manage pain. Refocusing is difficult, and patients may need frequent reminders.

Pain may also be modified by changing how the individual thinks about the pain. This can be accomplished by having the patient:

1. Think about the sensation being experienced not as pain but as a message to take a rest break.
2. Call the pain by a different name. This can sometimes make the person experience it differently, for example, as a tingling sensation rather than pain.
3. Periodically focus on the pain itself, but be aware objectively of how the pain changes over time.
4. Maintaining perspective on the pain is an important refocusing strategy. Patients often focus on their disabilities and lose sight of what they can do.

PAIN INOCULATION TRAINING

The inoculation approach to pain management involves helping the person prepare for the pain and decide how to handle the situation. It is based on a technique called *stress inoculation training* developed by Meichenbaum and his colleagues (Meichenbaum & Jarembo, 1982). The term *inoculation* is used because persons expose themselves to the pain in their imagination and practice handling it, so that when the actual challenge comes, they are prepared. To be fully conversant with this technique takes some extensive reading or actual training. The four basic components are described in Table 5-13, but the references by Turk et al. (1983) and Meichenbaum and Jarembo (1982) provide further information. The central feature of this ap-

Table 5–13 The Four Basic Stages of Pain Inoculation Training

Stage 1: Preparation

The person needs to prepare in advance for the pain before it becomes too strong. The person works to reject helplessness and maintain a positive attitude. Typical coping statements might include:

"I can deal with this pain."
"Of course, I'm a little depressed. That is expected. Let me focus on how I am helping myself."

Stage 2: Confrontation

The person uses the strategies planned to manage the pain. Negative emotions may accompany the pain, and these are confronted as well. Typical coping statements might include:

"This pain is getting bad. I'll practice relaxation and then call my friend."
"I won't get overwhelmed. I'll take it one step at a time."

Stage 3: Handling Critical Moments

The person may reach the point where he or she feels that the pain is overwhelming and that it is impossible to go on. Negative thoughts and feelings are often worse at these times. The person needs to accept the fact that the situation cannot be totally changed. However, specific approaches can make these difficult times bearable. Typical coping statements might include:

"I don't need to stop the pain totally, just get away from it a little."
"What I'm doing is not working. I'll switch to something else."

Stage 4: Reflection and Reinforcement

The person needs to reflect on how things went, congratulating the self for successes and planning modified strategies for the future. Often patients are not consciously aware of how they have modified their pain experience. Typical coping statements might include:

"I followed my plan pretty well. Next time I'll . . ."
"I am proud of myself for trying. I can't wait to tell my nurse."

proach involves developing positive coping statements to replace the negative thoughts and emotions that may accompany pain.

The goal of the pain inoculation approach is to help patients develop a plan for dealing with their pain. It is not just a set of positive phrases to say when they are in pain. Each stage must be individually fleshed out with the strategies described in this chapter. Patients must find what works for them and then practice their strategies. Incorporating the personal pain plan may be useful during the confrontational stage to help identify useful strategies.

Strategies Requiring Other Professionals

Rheumatic diseases are serious medical conditions that often involve considerable pain. The self-help strategies for pain management are not always sufficient. Referral to other resources is often necessary. The nurse may need to intervene with the physician to seek adjustments in medications. Other potential resources include occupational and physical therapists, pain clinics, mental health professionals, and self-help support groups. Experienced home health nurses know that making a referral is not always as easy as it may appear. Many patients slip through the cracks in the health care system. The principles for making a successful referral are reviewed in Appendix A to Chapter 1.

Medications

The drug treatment pyramid discussed in Chapter 2 has as its goal the control of inflammation and pain. First-line NSAIDs provide the cornerstone of management. Patients with rheumatoid arthritis follow a regular drug regimen, while those with osteoarthritis may take analgesic medication as needed.

Analgesics taken in addition to the prescribed regimen are preferably over-the-counter forms of aspirin, acetaminophen, or ibuprofen. Propoxyphene (Darvon) compounds may also be used for more severe pain. Because of the chronic nature of arthritis pain, every effort is made to avoid the use of narcotics, with their accompanying risks of tolerance and dependence. Short-term narcotic prescriptions may occasionally be necessary to control the pain of acute disease flare-ups, but they are restricted to oral agents in the lowest doses that will successfully control the pain.

Any medication regimen directed at the control of chronic pain is vulnerable to problems of over- or underuse. Patients may fail to take their medications and attempt to "tough it out" from fear of dependence, or they may unintentionally overuse their drugs in the quest for pain relief. The nurse plays an important role in assisting patients to integrate analgesic medications properly into their overall pain management program. The nurse establishes what medications the patient uses, both prescription and nonprescription, as well as the dose and the frequency of use. The nurse assesses the patient's knowledge about the medications and reinforces it as needed. Additional teaching should focus on the effectiveness of analgesics such as aspirin and acetaminophen, despite their inexpensive, over-the-counter status. Chronic pain is best managed by regular, routine drug administration, which allows therapeutic blood levels to be established and maintained, rather than waiting until the pain becomes unbearable. Stoic patients may need assistance to view analgesics as one aspect of a total self management program rather than as a symbol of defeat.

Local injections of intra-articular corticosteroids may also be used to control localized joint pain. The temporary use of systemic steroids will usually result in dramatic relief and is occasionally prescribed during acute disease flare ups. As discussed in Chapter 2, systemic use is strictly limited to avoid the severe side effects associated with prolonged steroid use. Empathetic teaching must be provided to help patients understand the necessity for restricting the use of this apparently effective therapy. Muscle relaxants may also be employed when muscle spasms add to the patient's joint pain.

Tricyclic antidepressants may also be ordered. They are often useful in chronic pain states where the effects of long-standing pain result in anxiety, depression, and sleep disturbances. Their use may also interfere with the production of pain-producing substances and assist the patient in regaining and maintaining control of the pain experience. The use of tricyclic antidepressants and their associated side effects are discussed in Chapter 7.

Physical Therapy

Physical therapy offers strategies that can be helpful adjuncts to pain management. Application of superficial heating modalities can raise the threshold for pain, increase superficial circulation, and facilitate muscle relaxation. Deep heat therapy can be provided through short-wave diathermy, microwave diathermy, or ultrasound to penetrate deeply into painful joints for pain relief.

Community health nurses may work with patients who are prescribed transcutaneous electrical nerve stimulation (TENS) devices for chronic pain management. TENS units deliver an electric current through electrodes applied to the skin surface over the painful area at trigger points or over a peripheral nerve. The pain relief produced by TENS is due to the mobilization of endogenous opiates and may be mediated by other pain transmission mechanisms that are not yet fully identified. The device may be prescribed for continuous or intermittent use. It consists of two or more electrodes connected by lead wires to a stimulator that is battery operated and about the size of a cigarette pack. The stimulator and wires can be detached for intermittent use, leaving the electrodes in place. Experimentation with different stimulators, electrode placement, and frequencies may be necessary to achieve optimum benefit. The nurse may need to reinforce teaching and provide support and encouragement for the use of this treatment. The patient will experience tingling, burning, or other paresthesias while the device is in place, and the voltage and rate of stimulation should be adjusted in response. The use of TENS is contraindicated for patients with cardiac pacemakers or a history of dysrhythmia.

All of these strategies require a complete physical therapy assessment. Strategies such as diathermy and ultrasound are unavailable in the home setting and require the patient to come to a hospital or clinic.

Psychologic Approaches

Biofeedback, hypnosis, milieu treatment programs, and support groups are examples of psychologic strategies that have been developed to meet the challenge of complex, chronic pain situations. While these strategies are not effective with all persons and do not totally eliminate the pain of arthritis, they may be useful for patients who, as a result of severe disease, poor adaptation, or lack of social support, require additional assistance in pain management. These strategies require the patient's commitment of time, energy, travel, and financial resources. The nurse needs to make it clear that these approaches offer no miraculous cures for pain but that they can assist patients to gain more control of their situation.

Biofeedback. Biofeedback involves teaching patients to use feedback from certain physiological processes (e.g., muscle tension, heart rate, peripheral temperature) to develop a physiologic state of relaxation and a mental state that allows them to cope with pain. Since the discovery in the 1970s that persons could be taught to gain control over certain physiologic activities, this process has been explored as a treatment for problems that may involve sympathetic nervous system arousal. Pain is often accompanied by sympathetic nervous system activation or muscle tension. Through the use of sensitive electrical equipment the patient can be taught to relax tense muscles; increase peripheral temperature, which indicates greater blood flow; or decrease a rapid heart rate or breathing.

Biofeedback can be useful in helping the person who has difficulty learning relaxation to master this skill. Research to date has not proven that biofeedback relaxation training is superior to general relaxation training. However, for some individuals, the equipment-based approach can provide the feedback that learning and relaxation are taking place. Biofeedback is also useful because it provides distraction from the pain and helps individuals feel that they have more control over their body. Since patients with arthritis may feel a loss of control over their bodies, this can be an important benefit.

It takes considerable training and practice to become an effective provider of biofeedback training. Before initiating a referral, the nurse should be certain that the providers are skillful and experienced in applying biofeedback techniques for the management of chronic pain.

Hypnosis. Hypnosis is a form of deep relaxation created by concentrating and focusing attention internally—away from one's usual thoughts or activities. Suggestions about positive changes and pain control seem more easily accepted and effective when the person is in this state. Modern hypnosis developed during the middle to late 1800s, when it was used in many cases to induce analgesia for surgical procedures. There has been a recent resurgence of interest in hypnosis as a pain control procedure. The ability to use hypnosis varies from person to person. The patients who appear to benefit most from hypnosis pain management are those who believe that it will help them and have ability in this area.

It is difficult to refer patients specifically for hypnosis. They may be poor subjects or greet the idea with skepticism. Referral to a pain clinic may, however, eventually result in the suggestion or use of hypnosis. Providing hypnosis treatment, as with biofeedback, requires both education and training.

Pain Clinics. Pain clinics are being developed in many areas, bringing together a multidisciplinary team to provide comprehensive treatment to persons with chronic pain problems. These programs are typically staffed by a team of health care professionals who specialize in the management of pain. Here the person may be enrolled in an inpatient or outpatient program designed to achieve pain control. Usually a number of simultaneous treatments are used. A milieu is developed in which the educational goal of pain management is emphasized, along with treatment.

Some persons with severe arthritis pain problems need this comprehensive service. Patients who are "doctor shopping," developing increasing dependence on narcotic analgesics, or becoming permanently disabled or dysfunctional due to their pain are candidates for this type of treatment. Referral from the primary physician or rheumatologist is usually required and always advisable. It is difficult to provide a comprehensive pain management program when patient care is fragmented and communication is poor. It is useful for nurses to identify pain management centers in their referral areas that can provide such services.

Support Groups. Most people feel that sharing experiences with a group of individuals who have similar concerns is helpful. The basic goal of arthritis or pain management support groups is to provide an opportunity for sharing feelings about arthritis and its related difficulties. A group may help the person feel understood, demonstrate that the person is not alone, and provide new ideas for coping with the arthritis pain. Social psychology research suggests that observing other persons modeling positive coping strategies is an effective way of learning new behaviors.

Groups may be run by professionals or by persons with arthritis. Some of them focus on pain control, while others have no specific focus but work on all aspects of arthritis. In addition to acquiring specific skills, the person may benefit from the socialization, helping others and enjoying the time spent outside the home. Potential sources of support groups are the local chapter of the Arthritis Foundation, senior citizens centers, pain clinics, or community hospitals. The community health nurse should be familiar with the support groups that are appropriate for arthritis patients in the area.

The management of pain is an important and ongoing aspect of arthritis care. Nurses have a vast array of strategies to suggest or employ with patients who are attempting to manage their care effectively.

Table 5-14 summarizes some of the basic comfort principles in care plan format. The key to success is to help the patient complete a personal pain plan and follow it.

Table 5–14   Care Plan for Pain Management

Nursing Diagnosis	Patient Goal	Intervention
Alteration in comfort: chronic pain related to the effects of increased disease activity.	Patient will increase knowledge of self-management strategies useful in chronic pain control.	1. Teach patient about the cause of arthritis pain and its challenges. 2. Explore with patient the relationship between stress, anxiety, and pain. 3. Assist patient to set realistic goals for pain management. 4. Introduce patient to various strategies for relaxation and cognitive pain management. Assist patient to select appropriate strategies for lifestyle. 5. Introduce patient and family to correct techniques for performing selected strategies.
	Patient will incorporate appropriate physical and mental strategies into daily activities.	1. Teach patient importance of compliance with prescribed drug regimen. Instruct patient in safe augmentation of regimen with over-the-counter analgesics. 2. Assist patient to coordinate daily activities to balance activity and rest. 3. Instruct patient and family in the safe use of home modalities for the application of heat and cold. 4. Instruct family in the safe use of massage. 5. Teach patient about proper positioning for rest—use of firm mattress or bed boards and avoiding pillows.

continued

Table 5-14 Care Plan for Pain Management (*Cont.*)

Nursing Diagnosis	Patient Goal	Interventions
		6. Assist patient to practice the relaxation or other cognitive strategies selected. Encourage and reinforce their use.
	Patient will express ability to self-manage arthritis pain.	1. Teach patient to intervene promptly in order to manage pain before it becomes unbearable.
		2. Encourage patient to develop and follow a personal pain plan.
		3. Teach patient appropriate pain inoculation techniques.
		4. Instruct patient to maintain log of activities, pain level, pain strategies used, and their effectiveness.
		5. Monitor the effectiveness of the patient's overall pain management program. If home-based strategies fail, refer patient for additional help as needed.
		6. Provide family with information about arthritis support groups in the area.

CASE STUDIES

1. Mrs. Martha Zimmer is a 72-year-old woman with severe osteoarthritis in her lower back. She has just been discharged from the hospital following a left total hip replacement. Her pain is present most of the time, but it also exacerbates unpredictably. Mrs. Zimmer is an otherwise healthy woman who is extremely energetic and deeply resents the intrusion of arthritis pain into her life. She is

determined not to "give in to it" and remains active from dawn to dusk with housework, church, and volunteer work and frequent entertaining. She rarely rests during the day and has few established leisure time activities.

Mrs. Zimmer uses no overall pain management plan. She dislikes pills and only resorts to an occasional Tylenol when the pain is unbearable. She often uses a heating pad or hot bath for soreness and reports that they do provide relief. The idea of massage for stiff muscles appeals to her, but she says that her husband's hands are too rough. Mrs. Zimmer admits to being a nervous person who suffers from insomnia. She is very involved with her children and grandchildren, and worries about them a lot. She is determined not to become incapacitated and a burden on her family.

1. What deficits are apparent in Mrs. Zimmer's approach to pain management?

2. Is any teaching indicated here concerning arthritis pain and its effects?

3. What personality characteristics could be used to assist Mrs. Zimmer to manage her pain more effectively?

4. What physical modalities might be effective in improving her pain management?

5. What relaxation strategies might be acceptable to her? What cognitive strategies might effectively complement her approach to life?

6. Does Mrs. Zimmer need any interventions or resources outside the home at this time?

2. Wendy Jeffers is a 36-year-old woman who was diagnosed as having rheumatoid arthritis a year ago. Her disease started severely and has not yet responded well to drug therapy. Pain, which is often acute, has been an ongoing feature of the disease thus far.

Wendy is frightened of both the disease process and the pain. She says, "I'm such a baby about pain. I try, but I just can't stand it." Wendy follows her drug regimen carefully and supplements it as needed with Tylenol and codeine. This only succeeds in making the pain bearable.

Wendy lives alone and admits that bad days cause her to take to her bed in tears. Rest is the only physical modality of pain control that she practices. She reports that she is most comfortable lying in bed with her painful joints supported on pillows. She has been withdrawing from social contacts more and more often. She considers herself bad company: "Who wants to spend time with someone who does nothing but whine about how much she hurts? I don't want to be this way, but how can I stop?"

1. What goals might be appropriate to set initially with Wendy concerning pain management?

2. What strategies might be appropriate in beginning to help Wendy reestablish control?

3. What teaching is needed in this situation concerning arthritis pain and its effects?

4. What physical modalities should Wendy try?

5. What relaxation or cognitive strategies might be helpful in assisting Wendy to control her pain?

6. Are there any resources or strategies outside the home that you feel would be useful to Wendy at this time?

PATIENT EDUCATION MATERIALS

Florence, D., Hegedus, F., & Reedstrom, K. (1982). *Coping with chronic pain: A patient's guide to wellness.* Sister Kenney Institute, Abbott-Northwestern Hospital, Publications—Audiovisual Office, 800 E. 28th St. at Chicago Ave., Minneapolis, MN 55407.

Swezey, R. L., Wegener, S. T., & Ziebell, B. A. (1987). *Coping with pain. The battle half won.* Arthritis Foundation, 1314 Spring St., N.W., Atlanta, GA 30309.

AUDIOVISUAL MATERIALS

Arthritis Foundation. (1980). *Coping with pain.* Arthritis Foundation—New York Chapter, 115 E. 185th St., New York, NY 10003.

Huycke, S. (1981). *Arthritis: A dialogue with pain.* National Film Board of Canada, 1251 Ave. of the Americas, New York, NY 10020-1173.

BIBLIOGRAPHY

Boguslawski, M. (1980). Therapeutic touch. A facilitation of pain relief. *Topics in Clinical Nursing, 2,* 27–36.

Bradley, L. A., Young, L. D., Anderson, K. O., McDaniel, L. K., Turner, R. A., & Agudelo, C. A. (1984). Psychological approaches to the management of arthritis pain. *Science and Medicine, 19,* 1353–1360.

Davis, M., Eshelman, E. R., & McKay, M. (1982). *The relaxation and stress reduction workbook.* Oakland, Calif.: New Harbinger Publications.

Donovan, M. I. (1980). Relaxation with guided imagery: A useful technique. *Cancer Nursing, 80*(2), 27–32.

Dudley, H. F., & Huskisson, E. C. (1972). Pain patterns in the rheumatic disorders. *British Medical Journal, 4* 213–216.

Heidrich, G., & Perry, S. (1982). Helping the patient in pain. *American Journal of Nursing*, *82*(12), 1828–1833.

McCaffery, M. (1979). *Nursing management of the patient with pain*, 2nd ed. Philadelphia: J. B. Lippincott.

Meichenbaum, D. H., & Jarembo, M. E. (eds.) (1982). *Stress prevention and management: A cognitive-behavioral approach*. New York: Plenum.

Meinhart, N., & McCaffery, M. (1983). *Pain: A nursing approach to assessment and analysis*. Norwalk, Conn.: Appleton & Lange.

Melvin, J. L. (1982). Joint protection and energy conservation instruction. In J. L. Melvin (ed.), *Rheumatic disease: Occupational therapy and rehabilitation* (pp.351–371). Philadelphia: F.A. Davis.

Mersky, H. (Chairman) and the IASP Subcommittee on Taxonomy. (1979). Pain terms. A list with definitions and notes on usage. *Pain*, *6*, 240–252.

Mohr, E. (1987). *The chronic pain control workbook*. Oakland, Calif.: New Harbinger Publications.

Mooney, N. E. (March–April 1983). Coping with chronic pain in rheumatoid arthritis. Patient behavior and nursing interventions. *Rehabilitation Nursing*, 20–25.

Moore, D. E., & Blocker, H. M. (1983). How effective is TENS for chronic pain? *American Journal of Nursing*, *83*(8), 1175–1180.

Olsson, G., & Parker, G. (1987). A model approach to pain assessment. *Nursing*, *87*(5), 52–57.

Pigg, J. S., Driscoll, P. W., & Caniff, R. (1985). *Rheumatology nursing. A problem-oriented approach*. New York: Wiley.

Rehabilitation through learning: Energy conservation and joint protection—A workbook for persons with rheumatoid arthritis: Instructor's Guide. NIH Pub. No. 85-2743). Washington, D.C.: U.S. Government Printing Office.

Riggs, G. K., & Gall, E. C. (1984). *Rheumatic diseases: Rehabilitation and management*. Boston: Butterworths.

Shealy, C. N. (1980). Holistic management of chronic pain. *Topics in Clinical Nursing*, *2*, 1–7.

Simpson, C. F. (1983). Heat, cold or both? *American Journal of Nursing*, *83*(20), 270–273.

Sternbach, R. (ed.). (1978). *The psychology of pain*. New York: Raven Press.

Turk, C., Meichenbaum, D., & Genest, M. (1983). *Pain and behavioral medicine. A cognitive behavioral perspective*. New York: Guilford Press.

Waletson, M. (1978). Hot and cold therapy. *Nursing*, *78*(10), 46–49.

Wegener, S. (June 1986). Relaxation strategies work for arthritis pain. A paper presented to the Arthritis Health Professions Association, New Orleans.

6

Fatigue and Sleep Disturbance in Arthritis

Stephen T. Wegener
Cynthia Stabenow Kulp

Fatigue and sleep disturbances are common problems in persons with arthritis. The problems may exist independently or may be closely interwoven. The experience of a restless or sleepless night can leave patients too tired to face the day, while chronic fatigue may cause patients to seek more rest and sleep, yet often not find relief. These problems may be severe and may interfere significantly with their preferred lifestyle. The link with chronic pain is also clear. Coping with pain on a daily basis drains the individual's remaining energy and yet may prevent or interrupt needed sleep. Each of the problems can aggravate the other.

FATIGUE

Fatigue is a complex, nonspecific phenomenon that frequently accompanies both osteoarthritis and rheumatoid arthritis. For patients with osteoarthritis, fatigue is a common result of coping with chronic pain and of the fact that normal activities require more effort when joints are painful and muscles are weak. These same circumstances apply to patients with rheumatoid arthritis, but in addition, this form of arthritis causes fatigue as a systemic manifestation of the disease. Its presence and severity are often regarded as reliable indicators of disease activity.

Assessment of Fatigue

The word *fatigue* evokes many meanings, depending on who is being asked. In persons with arthritis, this term frequently overlaps with *tiredness, lack of energy,* and *depression.* Patients with severe fatigue may substitute complaints of pain for complaints of fatigue, since they are more specific and less likely to be attributed to psychological sources. The nurse's assessment of fatigue therefore will often lack precision, but it can disclose other factors that may be contributing to the problem, such as anemia, muscle atrophy, sleep disturbance, or emotional stress. Table 6-1 presents some assessment questions that are specifically targeted at fatigue and can be incorporated into a more complete sleep pattern *or* activity pattern assessment. By its specific assessment, the nurse is validating the existence of arthritis fatigue and indicating her willingness to help the patient deal with the problem.

It may also be important to assess another dimension of the patient's activities in order to better understand the scope and impact

Table 6–1   Assessment of Fatigue

1. Do you have difficulty with tiredness or fatigue?
   _____ Yes   _____ No

   How long has fatigue been a problem for you? _____
   On a scale of severe/moderate/mild, where would you rank it? _____

   What time of day does it seem to be the greatest? _____

   (Record as number of hours between awakening and onset.)
   (Use average day involving typical activities.)

   Is your fatigue present upon sitting and reclining or only upon ambulation?
   Both? _____

2. Do you notice any relationship between your tiredness/fatigue and other
   problems you have with your disease? _____

3. Do you rest during the day?
   _____ Yes
       Describe how and length of time. _____

   _____ No
       Give reason. _____

   _____ How many hours/day do you spend in bed?

   _____ Do you feel refreshed after rest or sleep?
4. How do you do your work throughout your day?
   _____ Go from task to task until unable to continue

   _____ Alternate light and heavy work

   _____ Rest

   _____ Use energy-conserving methods

Source: Pigg, J.S., Driscoll, P.W., & Caniff R., *Rheumatology nursing*. Copyright © 1985 John Wiley & Sons, Inc. Reprinted by permission of John Wiley & Sons, Inc.

of fatigue. This dimension includes the value or meaningfulness of certain activities for the individual with arthritis. Fatigue affects relationships and the patient's social and family roles. When fatigue causes parents to say no to children's requests for activity or causes spouses to stop joining in shared social activities, the results may be much more important than the activity itself. Patients are not always consciously aware of how much of their time and energy are taken up with activities that have little or no value to them. Table 6-2 presents

Table 6–2 An Activity Record That Assesses Meaning and Value Associated with Daily Activities

Day 1 Half-hour beginning at:	Morning Activity	Question 1 During this time I felt pain	Question 2 During this time I felt fatigue	Question 3 I think that I do this	Question 4 I find this activity to be	Question 5 For me this activity is	Question 6 Others value this activity	Question 7 I enjoy this activity	Question 8 I stopped to rest during the activity
		1 = Not at all	1 = Not at all	1 = Very poorly	1 = Very difficult	1 = Not meaningful	1 = Not at all	1 = Not at all	1 = Yes
		2 = Very little	2 = Very little	2 = Poorly	2 = Difficult	2 = Slightly meaningful	2 = Very little	2 = Very little	2 = No
		3 = Some	3 = Some	3 = Average	3 = Slightly difficult	3 = Meaningful	3 = Some	3 = Some	
		4 = A lot	4 = A lot	4 = Well	4 = Not difficult	4 = Very meaningful	4 = A lot	4 = A lot	
7:00 a.m.	Wake up and shower	1 2 3 4	1 2 3 4	1 2 3 4	1 2 3 4	1 2 3 4	1 2 3 4	1 2 3 4	1 2
7:30 a.m.	Breakfast	1 2 3 4	1 2 3 4	1 2 3 4	1 2 3 4	1 2 3 4	1 2 3 4	1 2 3 4	1 2
8:00 a.m.	Exercise	1 2 3 4	1 2 3 4	1 2 3 4	1 2 3 4	1 2 3 4	1 2 3 4	1 2 3 4	1 2

Source: Activity Record (ACTRE) Bethesda, MD. Department of Rehabilitation Medicine National Institutes of Health Clinical Center, 1984. Used with permission.

an assessment tool for use with arthritis patients that taps the dimensions of meaning and value in activities performed.

Once this assessment is completed for a sample day or week, it may reveal that a large percentage of the patient's day is spent doing activities that are painful, fatiguing, worthless, and meaningless for the patient. This assessment can provide the basis for an intervention program with the arthritis patient who needs to choose among activities, ask for assistance with tasks, or direct other family members to do the job previously done by the patient.

A chronic disease like arthritis disrupts all of the patient's roles, habits, and behaviors of daily life. How the patient adapts to the disease may be partly due to the patient's *flexibility* in letting go of old habits, behaviors, routines, or responsibilities. The nurse can help patients understand that they have choices. The fact that patients have always done their own housework or yard work, for example, does not mean that these patterns of behavior must continue, particularly if they involve activities that the patient does not value. The nurse may serve as a catalyst, enabling the patient and family to make needed changes.

Management of Fatigue

The management strategies for fatigue overlap in many respects with the strategies discussed for pain and problems with daily living skills (see Chapters 3 and 5). They focus on pacing, energy conservation, muscle strengthening, and the management of stress. To complicate the problem of fatigue, patients with rheumatoid arthritis are also typically anemic. The anemia is usually mild and benign, but it can be another source of energy drain. The anemia of rheumatoid arthritis rarely responds to iron supplements, but ruling out iron deficiency anemia should be one of the basic interventions directed at the problem of fatigue.

Energy Conservation
Energy conservation and joint protection tend to be linked in the occupational therapy literature. Joint protection techniques help decrease pain in joints and allow patients to complete activities more comfortably, thus saving energy expended during painful activities. It is difficult for patients with arthritis to grasp the concepts of energy expenditure and energy conservation or storage. The nurse needs to convert these concepts into strategies for the patient at home. If an

occupational therapist is available, the two professionals can assist the patient to implement an energy conservation program at home that contains the three elements discussed below.

Planning Ahead. The patient should be encouraged to prepare a calendar or diary of activities for a week or two, circling periods of rest and activity. This encourages the patient (and family) to examine a week

Table 6–3 A Diary for Planning Activities and Rest

	Morning	Afternoon	Evening
Sunday	Prepare breakfast Dishes Rest break Church	Visit with family Rest break Prepare dinner	Rest break Church meeting
Monday	Prepare breakfast Dishes Laundry (one load) Rest break	Clean (1 room) Rest break Prepare dinner	Rest break Walk with spouse
Tuesday	Prepare breakfast Dishes Rest break Clean (one room)	Rest break Aquatics exercise Rest break Prepare dinner	Rest break Grocery shop
Wednesday			
Thursday			
Friday			
Saturday			

visually and set priorities regarding family jobs and activities. The nurse can assist the patient to assess the amount of pain or fatigue that follows this newly structured weekly plan. A chronic disease like arthritis demands *behavior* changes, and the nurse may need to work with the patient and family over time before evidence of behavior change is seen. Table 6-3 presents a sample activity planning diary.

Organizing and Arranging Space. The nurse and the patient can examine the home for optimal organization. Clutter requires extra cleaning and may cause the environment to be unsafe for patients ambulating with walkers or crutches. The nurse can examine a room during each home visit, making suggestions for safety and ease of movement. The nurse also needs to make sure that the phone, medications, and adaptive aids (e.g., reacher, raised toilet seat) are in

Table 6–4   Care Plan for Fatigue

Nursing Diagnosis	Patient Goal	Interventions
Activity intolerance related to pain, inflammation, or psychological stress of chronic illness.	The patient will analyze daily activities and develop activity/rest patterns that are consistent with abilities.	1. Assess presence and severity of fatigue in patient's life. 2. Assist patient to analyze daily activities and prioritize or value them. 3. Collaborate with patient to develop an individualized activity plan. 4. Involve spouse and family as appropriate in plans for activity modification. Encourage patient to use appropriate assistance. 5. Incorporate energy conservation and joint protection principles into daily routines. 6. Assist patient and family to organize or modify the home environment to reduce energy expenditures.

place. Many busy persons probably feel that they could profit from this intervention, but when a patient has decreased mobility or joint pain and fatigue, it is not a luxury but a necessity.

Sitting to Work. The principle of sitting to perform activities may be difficult for the patient to incorporate into cooking, bathing, or dressing, but it allows these tasks to be performed safely while the lower extremities and the back are supported. Once the environment is properly arranged (e.g., a bath bench in the shower or a stool in the kitchen), it is easier for the patient to practice this energy-conserving strategy.

The individual may not be willing or able to make all of the energy-saving lifestyle changes outlined. The goal is to educate the patient about fatigue and the strategies for managing it. The intervention program can begin simply, with one or two modifications, and expand as indicated by the patient's response. All of the energy conservation strategies mentioned are discussed in more depth in Chapter 3. Table 6-4 summarizes basic interventions for fatigue in a care plan format.

SLEEP DISTURBANCE

Persons with arthritis are more likely to have sleep disturbances than other individuals of similar age. The quantity and quality of their sleep may both be impaired by pain, stiffness, or psychological disruption. Sleep disturbance is a highly subjective and personal event. Each person develops idiosyncratic sleep habits and patterns that, when disturbed, are categorized by the individual as sleep problems. These problems may be particularly important when an individual's overall functioning is already impaired by other aspects of the disease (see Figure 6-1). Minimizing sleep disturbances therefore takes on

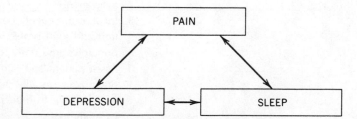

Figure 6–1. The relationship among sleep, pain and depression.

increased importance for persons with arthritis. Further, there is some evidence to suggest that sleep disturbances are related to exacerbations of disease activity. Successful prevention or treatment of sleep disturbances may contribute to overall control of the disease process.

The Sleep Cycle

A usual night's sleep is divided into sleep stages 1 through 4 and rapid eye movement (REM) sleep. Sleep stages are classified by electroencephalographic (EEG), electrooculographic (EOG), and electromyographic (EMG) patterns. Stage 1 is a transitory phase in which the person is moving from being fully awake to sleep. During this phase there is decreased EEG activity, EMG activity, and muscle tension. Persons usually report feeling relaxed and less aware of their surroundings. However, a person may report being awake, and it is during this stage that environmental noises may keep the person awake.

Stage 2 sleep is characterized by a further decrease in both EEG activity and muscle tension. For most persons, this is the stage in which sleep actually begins. It is followed by stage 3 and stage 4 sleep. These two stages are usually grouped together and are called *slow-wave sleep*. Brain waves continue to slow down and muscle tension continues to decrease. Stage 3 sleep is usually reached approximately 20–30 minutes after sleep begins. During stages 3 and 4 there is little movement; the person is deeply asleep and may be very difficult to arouse. Stages 3 and 4 sleep are thought to play an important role in physical restoration. Typically, the person passes briefly through stages 1, 2, and 3, followed by a long sojourn in stage 4.

After approximately 90 minutes, the person enters REM sleep. REM sleep, or *dream sleep*, is characterized by mixed EEG patterns similar to those of stage 1, with muscle tension at its lowest level. Rapid eye movements, which are associated with dreaming, are characteristic of REM sleep. Persons who are deprived of REM sleep tend to become hyperaroused, experiencing anxiety and other psychological disturbances. For this reason, REM sleep is thought to be involved with psychological restoration or "finishing the unfinished business of the day." It is also felt that REM sleep is important for learning and memory consolidation.

These four sleep stages occur in cycles each night. Typically, each cycle is approximately 90 minutes in duration, resulting in four to six cycles per night. Early in the night, stage 4 sleep is predominant. As the night progresses, the REM period grows longer and stage 4 decreases in length and frequency. The number of cycles depends on many variables, including age, previous sleep history, and medication. Some of these variables are important in the care of persons with rheumatic disease.

There is a decrease in stage 4 sleep with aging, and by the time a person reaches the sixth decade, it is almost totally absent from the sleep record. With aging, the time to the onset of sleep does not increase, but the person experiences less efficient sleep due to many more midsleep awakenings and a longer waking period at each occurrence. While this decrease in sleep efficiency is a general trend, there is a great deal of individual variability in sleep habits among the elderly. It appears that individuals who have chronic medical problems experience poorer sleep than those who are more healthy. Of course, those with chronic health problems such as arthritis can least afford to have poor sleep habits. It has been shown that poor sleep efficiency in persons with arthritis is related to higher levels of reported pain and depression. While causation cannot be established from the data available, it is clear that improved sleep should be an important goal in overall disease management.

A number of medications are also associated with drug-induced sleep disturbances. Drugs that may disrupt sleep, particularly in the elderly, include central nervous system stimulants, steroids, beta blockers, and bronchodilators. Individuals who are taking or being withdrawn from benzodiazepines may also experience sleep disturbances. The nurse should be aware of all medications the patient is taking and their potential to contribute to sleep disturbance.

Assessment of Sleep Disturbances

Sleep assessment seeks to determine if a sleep problem exits. There are several different types of sleep disturbances. The three most common types are sleep onset problems, sleep maintenance problems, and early morning awakening. Sleep onset problems are characterized by difficulty in falling asleep. Trouble falling asleep, either initially or later after sleep awakening, may be related to pain, inability to get comfortable, worry, or other factors. The nurse should pay special attention to anxieties or worries that may be keeping the patient awake. The typical person falls asleep approximately 5–15 minutes after lying down and closing the eyes, although as persons grow older, there is an increased variability in sleep onset time. In general, persons tend to overestimate the amount of time it takes them to fall asleep. Nevertheless, delayed sleep onset may be a problem for some individuals.

Waking up often during the night and having difficulty returning to sleep are the most common sleep disturbances in persons with rheumatoid arthritis. These problems are also a problem in other types of arthritis and are a common occurrence in the elderly. While it is unclear why these particular problems occur in these groups, the community health nurse should be alert to their occurrence.

Early morning awakening is often associated with depression or severe morning stiffness. While these are not the sole causes of this problem, they are the most common ones. The key to diagnosing this particular problem is to ask the patient whether he or she awakens earlier than usual or earlier than the preferred awakening time.

The assessment of sleep disturbances is relatively straightforward. In general, it is sufficient to ask the individual if sleeping is a problem. If the patient indicates that it is, it is important to obtain additional information regarding the type of sleep disturbance that is present. Often different types of sleep disturbances are grouped together under the rubric of "sleep problems." In order to develop an adequate treatment plan, it is important to know which problem is present. It is also useful to gather information on the solutions the patient has tried, how long the problem(s) have been present, and the patient's sleep habits and sleep hygiene. In some cases, it may be helpful to have the patient complete a daily sleep diary such as the one shown in Table 6-5. Using the sleep diary, the patient and the nurse can readily identify sleep problems of all three types, as well as any relationship to pain or mood changes that may be present. A sleep diary may be particularly helpful before, during, and after treatment to evaluate therapy. Patients often enjoy keeping track of their sleep habits, as this helps them understand their problem more clearly and allows them to be an active partner in the treatment process.

Potential Causes of Sleep Disturbances. Pain during the night is frequently cited as a cause of sleep disturbance in persons with arthritis. It can prevent persons from falling asleep and is cited as a reason for midsleep awakening. For most persons, particularly those with osteoarthritis, pain diminishes during rest and sleep. However, some persons complain that their pain increases at rest. This may be due to lack of distraction from the pain or to fatigue resulting from the

Table 6–5   Daily Sleep Diary

Instructions: Each morning when you wake up, answer the following questions about the sleep you had the night before and the pain from the previous day. Be sure to complete your diary every day.

	Mon	Tues	Wed	Thurs	Fri	Sat	Sun
1. Length of time to fall asleep (minutes).							
2. Number of times you awoke during the night.							
3. Did you awake in the morning earlier than usual? Yes or no							
4. Number of hours slept.							
5. Did you feel rested this morning? Very rested Rested Tired Very tired							
6. Were you satisfied with sleep? Very satisfied Satisfied Unsatisfied Very unsatisfied							
7. I took medication to help me sleep. Yes or no							
8. My mood yesterday was: 0 is very good or happy 10 is mood as bad as could be							
9. My pain yesterday was: 0 is no pain 10 is worst possible pain							

Source: S. Wegener, Ph.D. Sleep and Arthritis Project, 1985. All rights reserved.

day's activities. Morning stiffness may lead to early morning awakening.

Although pain and stiffness are readily identified as causes of sleep difficulty, there are other factors that also contribute to troubled sleep and should be considered as part of the sleep assessment. Several medicinal compounds may lead to sleep disturbances. The person's medications should be reviewed and potential problems identified and discussed with the physician. It is not uncommon for sleeping pills to worsen insomnia. Sleeping pills often decrease REM sleep and may make the person feel less rested the next day. Rapid withdrawal from sleep medication often leads to REM rebound and sleep disturbance characterized by nightmares, and is therefore not advised. Another potential problem is gastric distress related to NSAIDs. Often patients take these medications before bedtime to manage pain during the night. Occasionally this leads to gastric irritation and results in midsleep awakening. Another medical problem is nocturia. The incidence of nocturia increases with age and is often treatable by modification of fluid intake.

Psychological disturbances such as depression or anxiety are often related to sleep disturbances. Anxiety is more commonly associated with sleep onset and sleep maintenance problems, whereas depression is more often associated with early morning awakening. These adaptation alterations are not uncommon in persons with arthritis and often lead to sleep disturbance. It is important to assess what the person is thinking about while lying awake at night or having trouble falling asleep. Are there particular concerns, worries, or stresses that need to be identified and addressed? While persons are generally reluctant to identify psychological causes or other difficulties in their lives, they are often willing to link sleep disturbances to psychological causes. It may be during a discussion of sleep disturbance that the home health nurse becomes aware of significant worries or psychological disruptions.

As persons grow older, their sleep efficiency deteriorates. It is not uncommon for them to average 5–6 hours of sleep per night and awaken many times during the night. Older persons have less and less REM and stage 4 sleep, which may account for their feeling less rested in the morning. However, as long as they sleep more than 4 hours a night and feel rested, these changes should not be of particular concern. Patients may need education concerning normal sleep patterns for their age group.

Factors in the individual's environment such as noise, light, temperature, comfort of the bed, or bed partner's habits may all contribute to sleep problems. Each of these areas should be assessed. The person may be reluctant to express dissatisfaction with a bed partner's disruptive sleep habits such as snoring, moving about, or hours of bedtime. While these problems may appear relatively easy to address, they may in fact require assertive skills or material resources that are not available to the patient at this time.

Research suggests that irregular sleep habits due to rotating work schedules can contribute to sleep disturbances. Individuals with arthritis should be advised that regular sleep and rest periods are important in the management of their disease. Rotating shift work may contribute to exacerbation of their sleep problems and disease activity. Irregular sleep schedules should always be a concern in individuals who have sleep disturbances.

Sleep Hygiene

Basic sleep hygiene should be part of the education that the community health nurse provides to patients with sleep problems. While some of these ideas are common knowledge, it is surprising how many persons with sleep disturbances have not identified them. Encouraging the individual to consider personal sleep hygiene habits and how they may affect sleep is an important step in treating any sleep disturbance problem.

Regular Sleep Patterns. Maintaining a regular sleep schedule is a critical component in any sleep treatment program. Going to bed and waking up at the same time is useful in regulating the body's biologic clock and promoting better rest. While it is not important to maintain a strict schedule, a regular bedtime and rising time are critical first steps.

Exercise. Regular exercise has been associated with deeper, more restful sleep. Other sections of this book emphasize the need for persons with arthritis to perform daily exercise. This exercise will also contribute to good sleep patterns. Patients should be warned that exercise just before bedtime may arouse them, making sleep onset more difficult.

Eating and Drinking. In general, it is best to avoid eating large meals 1–2 hours before bedtime. Ingestion of large quantities of food, particularly in individuals with a hiatal hernia, is not advised, as it may lead to gastric problems. If the individual has difficulty falling asleep or staying asleep, it is advisable to avoid caffeine in the late evening. Caffeine is found not only in coffee but also in tea, chocolate, and a large number of soft drinks. Eating a small snack of crackers and milk while taking NSAIDs before bedtime may be useful in preventing gastric upset later in the night. Patients need to experiment with their eating and drinking habits to see what works best for them.

In general, persons should also avoid the intake of alcohol before bedtime, particularly those with midsleep awakening. Alcohol leads to sleep fragmentation later in the night and prevents a restful sleep.

Medications. Over-the-counter sleeping pills can contribute to sleep disturbances. Individuals who are taking these medications should consult with their physician regarding withdrawal and the need for appropriate treatment.

While education and sleep hygiene will not alleviate all sleep disturbances, education forms the basis for more extensive treatment. Further, education and good sleep hygiene may prevent the development of serious sleep problems in persons with arthritis.

Treatment of Sleep Disturbances

It may be helpful for individuals who experience joint pain during the night to take their NSAID or analgesic before bedtime so that they receive the benefit of these medications throughout the night. The physician should be alerted to the sleep problem and any changes in the medication schedule.

While the person with arthritis may require rest during the day, it is possible that long or frequent daytime naps will make sleep at night more difficult. Individuals with sleep onset problems in particular should be advised against taking extended naps in the late afternoon or early evening.

Pharmacologic Treatment. The most common medications used for sleep disturbances are hypnotics such as flurazepam (Dalmane), temazepam (Restoril), and triazolam (Halcion). Triazolam is useful for treatment of sleep onset insomnia but is less useful for improving sleep maintenance. This is due to its short half life of approximately 2–5 hours. It also loses its effectiveness over time, which restricts its use to short-term treatment. Temazepam is less efficient in inducing sleep but encourages sleep maintenance. Its half-life is approximately 8–13 hours. While it is not as effective in inducing sleep, it tends to remain effective over a somewhat longer period, up to 30 days. Flurazepam is useful in both inducing and maintaining sleep. This is due to its relatively long half-life of over 24 hours. It is effective for extended periods (30 days or more), although there is occasionally a hangover effect.

More recently, tricyclic antidepressants with sedative side effects have been used for the treatment of sleep disturbances and chronic pain in arthritis patients. These antidepressants are used in low doses of 10–75 mg. They are reported to have less effect on decreasing REM sleep and have little sedative effect the next morning. Further, they tend to maintain their sleep induction and maintenance qualities over extended periods. The most commonly used medications are amitriptyline (Elavil), doxepin (Sinequan), and trazodone (Desyrel). These drugs should be used cautiously with the elderly and with patients who have cardiac problems, as they produce frequent anticholinergic side effects, particularly cardiotoxicity. See Chapter 7 for a discussion of the side effects of tricyclic antidepressant drugs.

While pharmacologic interventions may play a major role in the modification of sleep disturbances in persons with arthritis, they are not the sole treatment. It is important that the individual take an active role in trying to alleviate sleep disturbances by following good sleep hygiene habits and perhaps involving themselves in one of the following behavioral treatments for sleep disturbances.

Behavioral Treatments

Research has shown that relaxation training is an effective way of modifying sleep disturbance in the general population. Relaxation training appears to be particularly useful when the individual is complaining of midsleep awakenings or attributes the sleep disturbances to tension, pain, or worry. In order to use relaxation training, it is helpful to identify the factors contributing to sleep disturbance that may be modified or alleviated by focused relaxation. Strategies for teaching deep breathing and relaxation are included in Chapter 5. Imagery has not been well established as a treatment for sleep disturbances. This may be due to the potentially activating effect of the images on the individual. Relaxation training, with its focus on deep breathing and muscle relaxation, is intuitively appealing to patients, as they consider the physiologic aspects of relaxation to be very similar to the physiologic state experienced when asleep. A relaxed state is conducive to falling asleep.

Changing Sleep Habits. If sleep onset is a problem, a technique developed by Richard Bootzin (Bootzin & Nicassio, 1978) called *stimulus control* may be particularly helpful. Bootzin hypothesizes that sleep

Table 6–6   A Six Point Stimulus Control Program for Changing Sleep Habits

1. *Go to bed only when you are sleepy.*
2. *Do not use the bed for any activity other than sleep. Sexual activity is the only exception to the rule.* If an individual spends a great deal of time in bed reading, eating, or watching television, the bed is no longer a cue for sleep onset.
3. *Once you go to bed, do not lie there awake for more than 15 minutes. Get up and go into another room. Return to bed only when you are sleepy.* This practice prevents individuals from tossing and turning in bed. While out of bed, they should pursue some quiet activity, such as reading, but avoid watching television or starting any project that encourages them to stay out of bed once they are sleepy.
4. *If you again cannot fall asleep within 15 minutes, repeat the previous step as many times as needed.* This is a difficult practice at first, but eventually it will improve the individual's sleep habits. During the first few nights, the individual may have to get out of bed four or five times.
5. *Set your alarm clock for the same time every morning and get up then, no matter how much or how little sleep you've gotten.* This establishes a consistent sleep pattern and prevents the individual from beginning to reverse nights and days.
6. *Do not take extended naps during the late afternoon or evening.* Adequate rest is essential in arthritis, but prolonged naps can discourage early sleep onset.

onset problems may develop in a number of ways. He believes, however, that these problems are maintained by losing the learned association between lying down in bed and falling asleep. The goal of this program is to help the person relearn this association. Stimulus control involves six major steps, which are outlined in Table 6-6. These points need to be carefully followed if the program is to succeed. The nurse should ensure that these instructions are available to the patient in written form.

The strategies for sleep hygiene, relaxation, and sleep habit changes are all readily available to community health nurses and are effective for many individuals with sleep disturbance. The nurse will involve the physician as needed through requests for medication prescriptions or adjustments. Individuals with severe sleep disturbances that persist in spite of these basic interventions should be referred for further workup. The basic interventions for sleep disturbances are summarized in Table 6-7 in a care plan format.

Table 6–7   Care Plan for Sleep Disturbances

Nursing Diagnosis	Patient Goals	Interventions
Sleep pattern disturbance related to pain and/or psychological disruption.	Patient will determine cause(s) of sleep disturbance.	1. Determine patient's normal sleep pattern. 2. Assist patient to complete a daily sleep diary. 3. Explore factors that may interfere with sleep and discuss with patient and family. 4. Discuss patient's medication schedule and its potential effect on sleep pattern. 5. Determine patient's normal daytime activity pattern.
	Patient will fall asleep promptly and experience increased periods of uninterrupted sleep.	1. Ensure that patient has a comfortable environment that is conducive to sleep onset. 2. Encourage patient to establish a regular schedule for sleeping and waking. 3. Encourage daytime activity and exercise, but promote relaxation before bedtime. Avoid late afternoon naps. 4. Teach patient to avoid heavy meals and alcohol before bedtime. Restrict evening fluids as necessary to prevent nocturia. 5. Teach patient proper use of sleep medications if indicated. Monitor their side effects and effectiveness. 6. Encourage patient to practice deep breathing ⇒

Table 6–7   Care Plan for Sleep Disturbances (*Cont.*)

Nursing Diagnosis	Patient Goals	Interventions
		and relaxation before sleep.
		7. Teach patient principles of a stimulus control program for modifying sleep habits if necessary.

CASE STUDIES

1. Penny Aston is a 42-year-old woman who has had rheumatoid arthritis for 4 years. She has had several disease exacerbations, although her disease is responding quite well to NSAID therapy. Penny is married and has four children aged 10 to 17. She has always been a full time homemaker, and her husband is a successful executive who travels often. They are financially comfortable and live in a large, modern home on an acre of land.

   Mrs. Aston's life is hectic, with housework, yard work, volunteer activities, and chauffeuring the children to multiple sports and social activities as well as serving as hostess for her husband's business entertaining. She has noticed that she is becoming increasingly fatigued, and there is tension in her marriage because she constantly seems to be too tired to keep up her former social pace. She is proud that she has made no concessions to her arthritis but is afraid that she may not be able to maintain her schedule much longer.

   1. How would you begin to attempt to help Mrs. Aston deal with her fatigue? What teaching might be indicated about fatigue and arthritis?
   2. What assessments are appropriate to help Mrs. Aston understand her activity pattern and its relationship to her fatigue?
   3. How can you assist her to set priorities in her day? How can she incorporate rest into her daily routine?
   4. What family education might be appropriate? What environmental modifications?

2. Joseph Dodd is a 68-year-old married man with osteoarthritis in his lower back and right knee. Recently, he reluctantly retired after 40 years of owning and running his own small business, as he had promised his wife that he would make time for them while they were still relatively healthy. He hasn't adjusted well to

retirement and is having trouble filling his day. He has no hobbies and spends his time puttering around the house and watching television.

Mr. Dodd is developing sleep problems for the first time in his life. He tosses and turns for hours trying to get to sleep, and then is awakened by the need to go to the bathroom and cannot get back to sleep. His back causes him much discomfort on sleepless nights. He often feels tired and naps frequently in front of the television during the day and evening. Fatigue is making him irritable, and Mrs. Dodd is beginning to wish that she had not encouraged him to retire.

1. What factors are probably contributing to Mr. Dodd's sleep problems?
2. What should be included in a sleep problem assessment?
3. Should Mr. Dodd be encouraged to ask his physician for any sleeping medications?
4. What basic strategies would you recommend to Mr. Dodd to help him deal with his sleep disturbances?

BIBLIOGRAPHY

Bootzin, R. R., & Nicassio, P. (1978). Behavioral treatment for insomnia. In M. Hersen, R. Eisler, and P. Miller (eds.), *Progress in behavior modification*, Vol. 6 (pp. 1–45). New York: Academic Press.

Clark, H. M. (March 1985). Sleep and aging. *Occupational Health Nursing*, *33*, 140–145.

Czeisler, C. A., Moore-Ede, M. C., & Coleman, R. M. (1982). Rotating shift work schedules that disrupt sleep are improved by applying circadian principles. *Science, 217*, 460–463.

Davis, M., Eshelman, E. R., & McKay, M. (1982). *The relaxation and stress reduction workbook*. Oakland, Calif.: New Harbinger Publications.

Demarest, C. (February 1986). Helping your patient get some sleep. *Patient Care, 20*, 61–71.

Dinner, D. S., Erman, M. K., Menn, S. J., & Morgan, J. P. (January 1986). An office workup for sleep disorders. *Patient Care, 20*, 20–38.

Furst, G. P., Gerber, L. H., Smith, C. C., Fisher, S., & Shulman, B. (1987). A program for improving energy conservation behaviors in adults with rheumatoid arthritis. *American Journal of Occupational Therapy, 41*, 102–111.

Hauri, P. (1979). What can insomniacs teach us about the functions of sleep? In R. Drucker-Colin, M. Shkurovich, & M. B. Sterman (Eds.), *The functions of sleep*, (pp. 251–271). New York: Academic Press.

Hayter, J. (1980). The rhythm of sleep. *American Journal of Nursing, 80*(1), 457–461.

Jestico, J. V. (1980). Night sedation and sleep. *Nursing, 80*, 886–888.

Meichenbaum, D. H., & Jarembo, M. E. (eds.). (1982). *Stress prevention and management: A cognitive behavioral approach.* New York: Plenum.

Melvin, J. L. (1982). Joint protection and energy conservation instruction. In J. L. Melvin, *Rheumatic disease: Occupational therapy and rehabilitation* (pp. 191–206). Philadelphia: F. A. Davis.

Ross, M. M., Hare, K., & McPherson, M. (October 1986). When sleep won't come. *The Canadian Nurse, 82*, 14–18.

Trubo, R. (1978). *How to get a good night's sleep.* Boston: Little, Brown.

Turk, C., Meichenbaum, D., & Genest, M. (1983). *Pain and behavioral medicine: A cognitive behavioral perspective.* New York: Guilford Press.

PART **4**

ADAPTATION ALTERATIONS

ADAPTATION ALTERATIONS

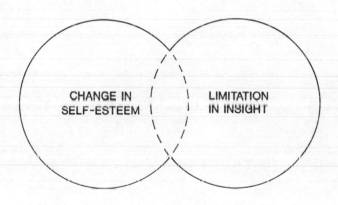

7

Psychological and Behavioral Aspects of Chronic Arthritis

Stephen T. Wegener

The chronic nature of arthritis requires the patient to make a number of lifestyle adaptations and alterations. Although the vast majority of patients adapt effectively, the potential for developing temporary or long-term psychological and behavioral problems secondary to the disease is very high. Several dimensions of chronic diseases differentiate them from acute medical conditions and make adaptation more difficult. Often in arthritis the cause of the condition is unknown. This uncertainty is a source of concern for both patients and health care professionals. A related problem is the unpredictability of the course and outcome of the disease. Some patients respond positively to treatment and maintain a high level of functioning, whereas others experience an unarrested downhill course leading to total dependence. This unpredictable course is stressful and can lead to feelings of hopelessness, depression, and inaction. Individuals with these cognitive and emotional characteristics may be overwhelmed by their disease and demonstrate poor adherence to medical regimens or increased disability.

The length of the illness also differentiates chronic arthritis from acute conditions. Individuals with arthritis often need to cope with pain and reduced functional abilities for the rest of their lives. This extended strain on personal, family, social, and financial resources often stresses these resources to the breaking point. These individuals need to develop coping skills and supports that will serve them for the duration of their disease.

The community health nurse can be of significant assistance to patients who are attempting to manage the psychological and behavioral aspects of their disease. The long-term goal is successful management within a framework of self-care. The community health nurse works closely with patients and families to identify problem areas and assist patients to develop the self-management skills and resources necessary to support optimal functioning. This process of nursing assessment and intervention, if successful, represents an active partnership between the nurse and the patient. Arthritis patients can sometimes be frustrating and difficult to work with, perhaps expecting the nurse to cure them or resolve their problems. But these patients also typically desire to maintain a high quality of life and participate fully in ADLs, and they bring this motivation to the nurse—patient partnership.

The major functions of the community health nurse are to provide ongoing nursing support, educate patients and families in the need for and purpose of self-management, teach patients self-help skills, and monitor their progress. The limitations of agency and patient resources are frequently an obstacle to patients' success in meeting their self-management goals. Being aware of the specific resources available in the local community is an essential task for the nurse. The nurse must also focus on the patient's goals rather than on her own. Patients differ greatly in the goals they set for managing their disease, as well as in the amount of help they will need or accept to achieve these goals. One individual may set relatively low goals for the self-management of the disease, whereas another may seek to maximize independent, active, self-management. Different individuals require varying levels of assistance to achieve these goals. The nurse must meet the patient within this context and avoid attempting to influence or alter the goal-setting process.

LEARNED HELPLESSNESS MODEL

The frequently encountered behavioral and psychological responses of patients to arthritis lend themselves to description and interpretation in terms of the learned helplessness model. Studies have shown that animals and humans, when placed in situations that are uncomfortable, negative, and uncontrollable, can develop a response pattern characterized by inactivity. When called on to respond in similar situations at a later time, they may be again unresponsive even if they are able to help themselves (Garber & Seligman, 1980). It is believed that both animals and humans learn when they cannot affect the outcome of a negative situation and therefore stop responding. This *learned helplessness* generalizes to other stressful events, and the individual acts helpless even when this response may not be appropriate. Depending on what and who the individual believes to be the cause of this helplessness, a number of problems may develop. These difficulties may include behavioral passivity, low self-esteem, and emotional changes such as anxiety and depression.

Figure 7-1 shows how the learned helplessness model may operate in patients with arthritis. The characteristics of arthritis are very similar to those that create learned helplessness in experimental situations. The person is confronted by a chronic disease with unpredictable flare-ups and remissions that may or may not be helped by medical intervention.

Some patients also bring to the chronic illness situation ways of thinking or limitations in insight that lead to negative beliefs. This

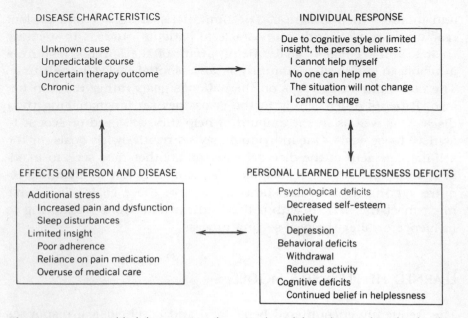

DISEASE CHARACTERISTICS

Unknown cause
Unpredictable course
Uncertain therapy outcome
Chronic

INDIVIDUAL RESPONSE

Due to cognitive style or limited
insight, the person believes:
I cannot help myself
No one can help me
The situation will not change
I cannot change

EFFECTS ON PERSON AND DISEASE

Additional stress
  Increased pain and dysfunction
  Sleep disturbances
Limited insight
  Poor adherence
  Reliance on pain medication
  Overuse of medical care

PERSONAL LEARNED HELPLESSNESS DEFICITS

Psychological deficits
  Decreased self-esteem
  Anxiety
  Depression
Behavioral deficits
  Withdrawal
  Reduced activity
Cognitive deficits
  Continued belief in helplessness

Figure 7–1. Learned helplessness is a theoretical model used to explain the development of psychological and behavioral adaptation alterations that accompany arthritis.

type of thinking facilitates such beliefs as "I cannot help myself" or "Arthritis is incurable, so there is nothing anyone can do." Learned helplessness is probably more likely if the individual believes that the situation is permanent and will not change.

These thoughts can lead to the learned helplessness deficits that are seen in the arthritis population. Psychological problems include decreased self-esteem, anxiety, worry, self-blame, and depression. These emotional disturbances facilitate the withdrawal and reduced activity that can follow the belief that arthritis is uncontrollable. The inactivity and negative emotional experiences tend to reinforce the belief that the patient is helpless. These patterns, in turn, maintain that belief, and the helplessness behaviors persist.

These learned helplessness deficits may have negative effects on both the person and the disease. The psychological deficits may create additional stress by increasing pain and sleep disturbance. The behavioral passivity may lead to poor adherence to the medical regimen or overreliance on passive coping responses such as taking pain medication. There is also the potential for either overuse of medical care services or the use of unproven remedies rather than self-management skills.

Many individuals with arthritis never develop this pattern of learned helplessness; instead, they bring to their arthritis experience what Rosenbaum (1983) calls *learned resourcefulness*. These individuals are often described as natural copers, survivors, or good problem solvers. They respond to the challenges of arthritis by taking an active approach, convinced that they have the ability to handle the challenges. How persons develop learned resourcefulness is uncertain. These individuals have an array of skills that can be used to control internal events such as thoughts, emotions, or pain.

Clinical examples of the concepts of learned helplessness and resourcefulness can be readily found. Disease flare-ups in rheumatoid arthritis are often accompanied by pain, swelling, limited ROM, and fatigue. One patient may perceive this situation as hopeless, unchanging, and beyond control. This person's attitudes and thoughts are characterized by statements such as "This will *never* change," "Arthritis is uncurable, *so nobody* can do anything," or "I am *totally* useless because I cannot do what I did in my job or around the house." These beliefs and attitudes easily lead to the negative emotions and behaviors that can accompany arthritis. Another patient, however, may perceive the situation differently as a result of upbringing, role models, or hardiness from unknown sources. This patient sees the negative situation as changing, controllable, and related only to the specific arthritis problems at hand. This person's attitudes and thoughts are characterized by statements such as "This phase will pass and I will feel better," "No one can cure my arthritis, but there are many other things I can do," or "My family and friends still like me even when I cannot do what I usually do." These beliefs characterize a learned resourcefulness approach and lead to active coping. The individual may still experience sadness, anger, and self-esteem problems, but they will probably not be as serious or enduring.

Ineffective individual coping and powerlessness are nursing diagnoses that may apply to arthritis patients at various times during their disease course. An ongoing nursing goal is to facilitate and develop an active, resourceful response to arthritis so that patients experience an increased sense of control over their lives. The nurse attempts to help the patient develop effective coping skills by teaching and modeling an attitude of learned resourcefulness.

Assisting Patients to Cope

The American Hospital Association's Health Education Project has described a two-level approach for assisting in the management of chronic disease (American Hospital Association, 1982). This general approach is useful in the community management of psychological and behavioral aspects of rheumatic disease and is consistent with a standard approach to nursing assessment and intervention. This approach is described as follows:

> The process being suggested is a step approach, similar to the familiar step approach used in drug therapy. Applying the process to an individual client, the provider introduces a first level strategy and evaluates the client's progress in self-management. If the first level strategy is unsuccessful with a client, a second level strategy is then introduced and evaluated. As the first step of designing such a protocol for a client population, providers need to identify a set of strategies that can be used with all clients initially. Second, providers need to identify a subset of more costly interventions which can be used with clients who have a history of poor adherence, who are having problems managing their condition, or who expect to have problems. (p. 4)

Some examples of first-level strategies that may be useful in helping arthritis patients develop self-management skills are outlined in Table 7-1. The nurse will determine which interventions are appropriate for a specific patient situation based on a careful assessment of the patient, family situation, and availability of local resources. A combination of strategies may be superior to a single approach.

After selecting initial strategies to help manage the identified problems, monitoring of the patient's progress is essential. As with hypertension treatment, in which regular blood pressure recordings are

Table 7-1   Level 1 Strategies for Persons with Arthritis

Home Visit Schedule	Examples of Strategies
Weekly visits until condition is regulated; biweekly visits for monitoring	Identify and use patient's goals as source of initial effort to increase motivation.
	Tailor regimen to patient's need and education.
	Educate about arthritis and rationale for management.
	Monitor quality of life, level of functioning (ADL and psychological).
	Involve family (as patient and family desire)
	Consider informal contracts regarding patient's behavior.

necessary to gauge the effectiveness of treatment, regular monitoring of functional and ADL abilities, compliance, depression, and social isolation is critical to treatment success. If level 1 strategies are not successful, additional efforts are necessary to assist the patient to manage the disease and develop self-management skills. Research has indicated that individuals with a history of non-compliance, poor memory, complex treatment regimens, or a complicated medical course are more likely to need additional help (Haynes, Taylor, & Sackett, 1979). If the nurse suspects that a patient may experience these difficulties, she should ask. Patients are the best and most reliable judges of their own behavior in the majority of cases.

With most patients, level 1 strategies are sufficient. However, when they have failed, or when the nurse suspects that difficulties may arise based on the profile described above, she may elect to use level 2 approaches. Some examples of level 2 strategies are listed in Table 7-2.

One goal of this approach is to assist the community health nurse to maximize the use of her own resources by focusing additional efforts only on those patients who require or request more services.

The success of these nursing interventions will depend to a large extent upon the relationship established with the patient. This basic maxim is true in all health care situations but is particularly important in the management of chronic disease in the home environment. Trust, honesty, and acceptance are hallmarks of the successful

Table 7–2   Level II Strategies for Persons with Arthritis

Home Visit Schedule	Examples of Strategies
Increase frequency of home visits	Consider simplifying treatment regimen.
	Assess patient's priorities and barriers that may affect self-management.
	Consider written patient contracts.
	Teach record-keeping skills.
	Consider education-support groups.
	Involve family more intensely (if both patient and family are willing).
	Use reminders (postcards, telephone).
	Refer for additional professional involvement (physical therapy, occupational therapy, mental health).

Table 7–3 Care Plan for Patients Experiencing Difficulties in Coping

Nursing Diagnosis	Patient Goal	Nursing Intervention
Powerlessness related to the illness, the treatment regimen, or a lifestyle pattern of helplessness.	Patient will experience an increased sense of control over daily activities and life situation.	1. Provide opportunities for patient to express feelings about self and disease. 2. Encourage patient to set own goals and help develop strategies for reaching them. 3. Provide appropriate positive reinforcement. 4. Teach patient to monitor own behavior and responses. 5. Encourage appropriate involvement of family
Ineffective individual coping related to the situational stressors of arthritis.	Patient will use self-management skills to complete everyday tasks. Patient will demonstrate increased functional activity	1. Assist patient to explore and evaluate usual coping pattern. 2. Assist patient to increase skills through role playing. 3. Provide appropriate positive feedback for behavior. 4. Teach appropriate self-help skills. 5. Make referrals as indicated to community agencies.

nurse–patient relationship. This means that the nurse must be open and honest with the patient regarding the disease process and prognosis, the patient's behavior, and the limits of the nurse's resources. It also requires acceptance of the patent's limited goals and resources. Both the nurse and the patient may be dealing with the disease and its related problems for an extended period of time. If the nurse–patient relationship is carefully established and maintained, self-management skills can grow and referrals to other professionals can be accepted. Table 7-3 summarizes in a care plan format the interventions appropriate for patients who are experiencing learned helplessness.

PROBLEMS RELATED TO CHANGES IN SELF-ESTEEM

The behavioral, psychological, and psychosocial adaptation alterations that accompany arthritis are related to the chronic nature of this condition. The problems encountered here are similar to those experienced by individuals with diabetes, multiple sclerosis, and muscular dystrophy. In addition to the stresses and changes in functional abilities experienced by these patients, the individual with arthritis has to deal with pain. The arthritis-related psychosocial problems often encountered by community health nurses include depression, anxiety, changes in body image/self-esteem, and disruption of roles (Anderson et al., 1985). Pain is such a major problem for patients with arthritis that its management is addressed individually in Chapter 5.

Depression

Depression is perhaps the most common emotional problem faced by all persons. Individuals with arthritis are at risk for developing depression in the course of their illness. Research findings consistently document a significant prevalence of depression in persons with rheumatoid arthritis and other chronic diseases (Cassileth et al., 1984). Most authors suggest that depression is a reaction to the experience of a chronic illness. It is not surprising that this population has a relatively higher incidence of depression. Depression may be conceptualized as resulting from a loss of positive experiences in the individual's life. A number of factors may contribute to this situation. Individuals with arthritis often experience decreased functioning leading to a loss of social roles, decreased participation in social events, and decreased financial support. Due to their illness, they are confronted with a loss of control over their lives and decreased life choices. As described earlier, this situation can lead to cognitive and behavioral changes associated with depression and feelings of helplessness/hopelessness and inactivity. Patients may become socially isolated or may manifest a variety of behaviors indicating a failure to cope adequately.

There are three general classes of symptoms associated with depression—changes in mood, changes in cognition, and physiologic disturbances. Depression is usually marked by a negative mood including feelings of sadness, loneliness, boredom, being unloved, guilt, or hopelessness. These feelings may be accompanied by crying or occasional displays of anger. The patient may describe these feelings directly, or they may be inferred from the patient's behavior. A stoic facial expression, speaking in a low tone, avoiding eye contact, becoming disinterested in one's personal appearance, or demonstrating little interest in activities are all potential signs of depression that should be noted.

Another central feature of depression is negative thoughts or a change in cognitive functioning. The change may be characterized by poor concentration, thought blocking, or the inability to complete a sentence. These individuals may also express negative thoughts concerning themselves, the future, and life in general.

The third cardinal feature of depression is a change in physiologic functioning. Typical signs include alterations in appetite, sleep patterns, or level of sexual energy. The nurse must be cautious in interpreting physiologic changes, as they may be a result of the disease process itself and not related to depression. Pain may modify the patient's willingness to participate in sexual activity, or medication may lead to appetite changes. It is critical to ask if the patient is interested in but unable to participate in these activities, rather than having lost the desire or interest. While arthritis patients may experience sleep disturbances, particularly an increased number of mid-sleep awakenings, the most common sleep disturbance occurring with depression is early morning awakening with an inability to return to sleep. (For more information on sleep disturbances in arthritis, see Chapter 6.)

If a nurse suspects that a patient is depressed, she needs to inquire into these symptoms in order to differentiate depression from the fatigue and pain associated with the disease. If changes in mood are found without accompanying symptoms in the areas of cognition or physiologic functions, intervention strategies in the home may be helpful once suicidal ideation is ruled out. If suicidal ideation is noted, or if mood changes are accompanied by cognitive or physiologic signs, a referral to a community mental health clinic or local hospital is appropriate. Patients with arthritis do not commonly become suicidally depressed, and high rates of suicide have not been documented in this population. Depression may, however, prevent participation in self-care and overall disease management. Often the community health nurse is in the best position to identify this problem and provide treatment recommendations.

Basic nursing interventions for depression include education, informal contracts, and promoting social involvement with supportive persons. Education regarding the signs and symptoms of depression helps patients recognize their condition, which is the first step in management. This education gives patients permission to express their negative thoughts or emotions and allows the nurse to normalize this experience as one that may accompany arthritis. Informal contracts to keep positive event diaries, participate in social events, or attend a local support group may also be helpful. Informing the family and significant others of the situation to encourage social activities and prevent isolation may provide the patient with more opportunities to experience positive events and rewarding social roles. A useful resource is *Feeling Good* by David Burns (1980), which is listed in the Bibliography. This volume on depression and self-management techniques describes a number of strategies that may be useful for community health nurses. Table 7-4 shows a form developed from one such strategy—the positive events diary. Often health care professionals focus on trying to isolate the cause of the depression—pain, social isolation, fear of further disability, loss of meaningful employment—in the hope of ameliorating the cause. While this can be a useful strategy, it is equally important to begin some active treatment in order to provide the patient with hope. This is particularly important with arthritis, as the cause of the depression is often difficult to identify and even harder to change.

If the depressed mood continues unabated or is accompanied by the other categories of symptoms, additional strategies need to be promptly employed. These strategies focus primarily on following through with the referral process and monitoring progress in treatment. The risk of suicide must be considered and regularly evaluated

Table 7–4   Guidelines for Developing a Positive Events Diary

Goal: To reacquaint yourself with the positive events in life that may be overlooked when you are depressed.

1. Write down at least one unplanned positive event that occurs each day. You
may write down as many as you chose. Examples: a phone call from a friend,
an accomplishment at work. Events do not need to be dramatic. Most of us
take pleasure from daily activities.
2. During week 2, try to plan at least one positive event for each day. Keep
recording unplanned positive events.
3. Review the diary with your nurse. Reinforcing positive events directs your
attention to them.

Sample Diary

Date	Event	Positive Thought or Feeling
8/9	Visited with children.	Realized they still care.
8/10	Received letter from Laura.	I haven't heard from her in a long time. I want to write back.
8/11	Tried a new recipe—success!	Family likes my cooking—their praise feels so good.
8/12	Finished new filing system at work.	Nice words from Mr. Jones. My hands are slower, but my brain isn't!
8/13	Made weekend shopping list.	Maybe I'm finally getting organized. I know it saves energy.
8/14	A wonderful night's sleep.	Makes the whole day better.

whenever severe depression persists. The nurse should not hesitate
to refer patients for more direct assistance whenever suicidal ideation
appears. Table 7-5 summarizes these interventions.

Some individuals with medical conditions such as arthritis are
reluctant to use mental health resources, as this implies that they are
mentally ill or that the pain is "all in their head." They need to be
made aware that depression may accompany arthritis and that mental health professionals can help them cope better with their disease.
Treatment may include counseling and/or medication. The most common medications used are the tricyclic antidepressants such as amitriptyline (Elavil) and imipramine (Tofranil). The use of these drugs is

Table 7-5   Level II Strategies for Depression Management

Make referral to mental health resources.
Monitor for self-destructive ideation, impulses, or behavior.
Monitor referral process to ensure that patient made contact with provider.
Promote compliance with mental health treatment regimen.

associated with a high incidence of anticholinergic side effects among others summarized in Table 7-6. In the elderly these side effects may be particularly problematic. The community health nurse should be alert to these problems, as they may be life-threatening or at least lead to poor compliance with the medication regimen.

Table 7-6   Tricyclic Antidepressants and Common Side Effects

Drug	Common Side Effects
Imipramine (e.g. Tofranil)	Central nervous system: drowsiness, sedation, insomnia, confusion
Amitriptyline (e.g. Elavil): greater anticholinergic and sedative effects than imipramine	Cardiovascular: orthostatic hypotension, ECG changes
Amoxapine (e.g. Ascendin): less cardiac toxicity than other tricyclic antidepressants	Gastrointestinal: dry mouth, constipation, increased appetite, taste bud changes
Desipramine (e.g. Norpramin): commonly causes confusion in the elderly	Eyes, nose: nasal congestion, dry eyes
Doxepin (e.g. Sinequan): greater sedative effects than other tricyclic antidepressants	Genitourinary: decreased vaginal lubrication, urinary retention, decreased libido, impotence
Maprotiline (e.g. Ludiomil): significant sedative effect	
Nortriptyline (e.g. Aventyl): less sedative and anticholinergic effects than imipramine but high incidence of confusion in the elderly	
Protriptyline (e.g. Vivactil): less sedative effects, but greater anticholinergic effect and cardiac toxicity than other tricyclic antidepressants	
Trimipramine (e.g. Surmontil): moderate anticholinergic effects but strong sedative effect	

Anger and Hostility

Some patients with arthritis experience anger as a result of being frustrated with difficult aspects of the disease process. Often these feelings are expressed in the question "Why me?" or anger may be expressed as hostility toward caregivers and family members. Expression of anger by the patient is often awkward for those with whom they come in contact, as it is difficult to know how to respond. Our society is generally more comfortable with the expression of depression or withdrawal than with anger and hostility.

The primary techniques available to the community health nurse for the management of anger are acceptance and active listening. Accepting this emotion without responding with withdrawal or anger in return is difficult. The nurse's recognition of anger as an appropriate and natural response to arthritis, or to any loss, is the key to acceptance. Active listening is an appropriate response to hostility expressed by the patient. It is usually not possible to talk the patient out of being angry, but listening often has a calming effect. The willingness to listen communicates acceptance of the individual and allows patients to ventilate these difficult feelings in a safe environment. These are all basic level 1 strategies that can be helpful in many situations. Usually these strategies are sufficient in the majority of cases, but occasionally patients are so hostile that they disrupt their interpersonal relationships. Referral for family or marital counseling is the appropriate intervention in this situation.

Anxiety and Other Negative Emotions

Many clinicians report high levels of anxiety, worry, and guilt in patients with arthritis. Research, however, has not confirmed that these emotions and experiences are more common in persons with arthritis than in other persons with chronic diseases. These findings may be the result of the multiple stressors of arthritis—changes in ADLs, increased medical expenses, changing roles, and chronic pain. In addition, the unpredictability of some forms of arthritis, notably rheumatoid arthritis and systemic lupus erythematosus, contributes to the development of these negative coping patterns. Anxiety and worry are signs of the helplessness that can result from being in an uncontrolled situation. These emotions may prevent the individual from following through on a treatment or rehabilitation program and thus can be major problems for the community health nurse.

Guilt and anxiety can be viewed as emotional/cognitive experiences that distract patients from the present, here-and-now reality. Guilt focuses on the past. What should have been done or not done, said or not said, thought of or not thought of, are all the focus of the individual captured in the past, dwelling on guilt. Individuals with arthritis have many opportunities to turn to guilty thoughts. They may not be able to fulfill certain roles at times—homemaker, worker, lover, or caretaker—and therefore have negative events to focus on. Anxiety focuses on fear of the future, and there are many negative events to anticipate with arthritis—potential disability, expenses, deformity, and ongoing pain. Anxiety and the accompanying cognitive component, worry, can keep patients preoccupied with difficulties in the future.

These emotional states have several negative consequences for anyone, but they may be particularly difficult for patients with arthritis. This emotional arousal is associated with increased sympathetic nervous system activity, including increased heart rate, blood pressure, muscle tension, and shallow breathing. This physiologic stress response puts additional strain on a body that is already dealing with a disease process. Further, there is evidence that individuals with these emotional and physiologic states have the perception of increased pain and a lower pain threshold. These emotional conditions can impede adherence to a treatment program, in addition to interfering with family and interpersonal relationships.

A central feature of these emotions and their related thoughts is the focus on either the past or the future. One way to help patients deal with these negative emotions is to encourage them to focus on the present. Trying to talk a patient out of anxiety or guilt is often ineffective. Basic level 1 strategies include education, family involvement, and informal contracting, but there are a number of other options. Patients should be made aware that they can change their behavior. They do not have to dwell on the past or worry about the future. Respect for patient autonomy means that patients have the right to continue on this course if they wish, but they should at least be aware of what they are doing. The nurse might offer some alternative strategies. If the patient exhibits readiness, the nurse might outline an informal contract in which the patient commits himself to begin working immediately on worries and anxieties.

Zeibell (1981) presents a six-step process to help patients cope with anxiety and guilt in the present:

Step 1. Have them identify exactly what they are worried about.

Step 2. Ask them to identify if there is anything they can do now to deal with the problem.

Step 3. If yes, set up a plan and assist them to do it.

Step 4. If no, ask what the guilt or anxiety is accomplishing.

Step 5. Assist them to deliberately let go of the guilt or anxiety. Encourage them to think of something they can do now to make themselves feel better. This may be something as simple as reading the paper or fixing a meal.

Step 6. Have them repeat the exercise several times per day. (p. 52).

Anxiety may be tied to fears of the inability to handle future events. Patients may benefit from listing the strengths and resources available to them and regularly reading the list. While these techniques are relatively simple and will not ameliorate incapacitating anxiety, they foster a model of self-help and active coping, which is extremely important. If the nurse recommends these techniques to a patient, it is critical that she follow up, just as she would for a medication prescription. If these skills are not followed up and reinforced, it is unlikely that the patient will continue to practice them. Encouraging the family not to respond continually to these negative emotional states, but instead to respond with encouragement to do something positive now, will also reinforce the message for the patient.

Changes in Body Image

Alterations in body image and self-esteem can be important sources of the negative emotions discussed above. These negative changes may result from modifications of social roles, loss of control, potential dependence, or alterations in body image that can occur with the disease. Changes in body image may be a particular concern with arthritis as compared to other chronic diseases due to the number of potential outward manifestations of the disease. Arthritis can lead to alterations in appearance due to joint deformity, alopecia, skin rashes, cushingoid features, or scarring from surgery. For some individuals, the use of assistive devices such as splints or walkers are negative events construed as insults to appearance or independence and therefore threatening to self-esteem. These concerns may not be verbalized by the patient but may take the form of poor follow-up in the use of recommended devices. Other signs of this problem may be self-imposed social isolation or the use of self-deprecating statements regarding the patient's appearance.

Table 7-7 Care Plan for Patients Experiencing Changes in Self-Esteem

Nursing Diagnosis	Patient Goal	Nursing Intervention
Disturbance in self-concent: Self-esteem related to disease effects and personal vulnerability.	Patient will participate in recommended therapies. Patient will set appropriate goals for self-management	1. Assist patient to identify assets and use strengths. 2. Assist patient to verbalize feelings. Use active listening and accept patient. 3. Monitor the extent to which the family influences patient's self-perceptions. 4. Teach family about their influence and how to affect the patient positively. 5. Establish contract for meeting short term goal.
Anxiety related to threat to role functioning.	Patient will experience reduced anxiety. Patient will focus on the present rather than the future.	1. Assist patient to identify and verbalize specific sources of stress. 2. Explore coping mechanisms and evaluate effectiveness. 3. Provide factual information about disease and treatment. 4. Assist patient to focus on day-to-day management.

continued

Table 7-7 Care Plan for Patients Experiencing Changes in Self-Esteem (*Cont.*)

Nursing Diagnosis	Patient Goal	Nursing Intervention
Disturbance in self-concept: body image related to changes in body structure and function.	Patient reconciles self-concept to changes produced by arthritis. Patient speaks positively of self.	1. Assist patient to identify and maximize assets 2. Encourage patient to maintain social contacts and involvement. 3. Explore availability of support groups in the community. 4. Encourage use of assistive devices as appropriate to support family and employment role performance. 5. Assist patient to role-play difficult social situations.

Many of the strategies that are helpful in managing depression are also useful in dealing with changes in self-esteem. Techniques that bring the patient's abilities and retained roles into focus are particularly helpful. These strategies include making a list of attributes or a positive events diary and participating in social support groups. Participation in social activity groups, whether designed specifically for patients with arthritis or communitywide, can be useful in treating social isolation or other symptoms of poor self-esteem. The Arthritis Foundation may be helpful in providing a list of local support groups or self-help classes.

Negative emotions and changes in self-esteem may be incapacitating in some individuals or may be related to clinical depression. Referral for in-depth mental health assistance as outlined in the section on "Depression" becomes the appropriate nursing intervention in these situations. Table 7-7 outlines the general interventions for patients with changes in self-esteem in a care plan format.

LIMITATIONS IN INSIGHT

A number of factors can influence the individual's ability to accept the disease, learn methods to manage it, and apply the acquired knowledge, methods, and skills. The individual is faced with an onslaught of new knowledge and the need to practice many new health care behaviors while adjusting to a painful and unpredictable medical condition. It is not surprising that some individuals demonstrate limitations in insight, as described by Pigg, Driscoll, and Caniff (1985). These authors suggest that limitations in insight may be due to the chronicity of the disease, a lack of readiness to manage it, or a paucity of knowledge and skills. The modern medical system has led many persons to believe that all diseases and conditions can be treated and cured. It takes time for patients to accept the unremitting nature of arthritis. When in a state of disbelief, they are not prepared to absorb new information or practice new skills. The acceptance process takes time, but the majority of patients succeed. Some individuals, however, choose to use denial or avoidance as their major coping strategy. These are defense mechanisms that protect self-esteem from threats that are either real or perceived. For some persons, acceptance of the chronic nature of their disease implies accepting a life of pain without the ability to perform many of the roles and activities that are rewarding to them. This denial can lead to avoidance of new learning and management skills that could alter the course of the disease. This denial can be accompanied by inactivity, depression, and withdrawal.

Limitation in insight leading to poor adaptation may also be related to other environmental or personal variables. Limited intellectual resources, poor reading or writing skills, and the discomfort associated with the disease may all negatively influence the individual's ability to respond to teaching or other nursing interventions. An assessment of these factors is important when planning a treatment program for an individual.

Patient education is a major role of the community health nurse. An understanding of the disease process is the basis for other levels of treatment and may facilitate adjustment to the changes required by the arthritis. Knowledge is power. In a situation where individuals potentially feel out of control, as if their body has rebelled against them, an understanding of their condition can be extremely important. It is, of course, impossible for newly diagnosed patients to develop physical or psychological coping strategies without an understanding of what their options are. Providing information on medication, pain management techniques, potential surgeries, or clarifying misconceptions is the first step in overcoming limitations in insight.

Family Influences

In addition to qualities of the individual that may influence the readiness to adapt and cope with arthritis, the social and family environment can either reinforce or discourage positive adaptation. A nursing assessment of the family environment is critical. The community health nurse is in an ideal position to observe patient–family interaction. She has access to the family both in gathering information and in initiating interventions. While she is in the home, the reaction of family members to the patient's complaints, needs, and illness can be directly observed.

Families, like individuals, have different reactions to the presence of arthritis in their lives. Some families adapt appropriately, while others exhibit less helpful responses. Reactions can range from disbelief (disallowing the individual's problems, as there is no outward manifestation of disability), to overreaction (including fulfilling the person's every need). Changes in employment, homemaking, leisure, or sexuality that may be required of the person with arthritis demand changes in the family system. How the spouse, children, other family members, and friends respond to these changes will strongly influence how the individual copes with the disease and its limitations.

Family and friends are powerful resources that can be used by the community health nurse. These resources need to be assessed and guided in the proper direction. An assessment of how the patient's family and friends respond to the disease is important. This assessment is similar to that conducted with the patient, although it may not be as formal. Observation and a few questions replace a thorough examination. Areas to be assessed include the family's knowledge of the disease, the treatment, and the prognosis. Are the family members aware of the patient's changing abilities? Do they know what they can do and what they should refrain from doing? The unpredictable nature of many types of arthritis makes adjustment and management difficult. The spouse and other family members may respond to the disease as if it were an acute illness and encourage extended bed rest or inactivity. They may take over the patient's family responsibilities or treat the patient like an invalid. This behavior, which is appropriate in acute illness, can have negative effects on all family members. The patient may come to feel useless, with no roles to perform, and inactivity can lead to a further decline in health. Family members may become angry about the additional work that has been "forced" on them. Here basic interventions centering on education and informal contracting can be useful. These families require education about the chronic nature of the disease and the need for continued activity on the part of the patient. Helping the patient or the family to negotiate shared responsibilities within the limitations of the disease and yet allow the patient to retain important role functions is critical. Other families may not recognize the need to adapt to the limitations imposed by the illness. Spouses may expect work, homemaking, or sexual activity to return to normal after a brief period. These families require education concerning the limitations imposed by the disease and the need for change in response to the illness. Here the community health nurse may need to encourage assertive behavior on the part of the patient or help facilitate an understanding of the patient's changed abilities and roles. Attendance at meetings of arthritis self-help or support groups by the patient and spouse may be helpful in addressing these concerns.

Most spouses and families can make these adjustments independently or may require, at most, basic interventions using education or informal contracting. However, marital relationships or families that were marginally dysfunctional before the onset of arthritis may need more help. Appropriate interventions may include formal contracting and referral for outside help at a community mental health clinic or family guidance center. A careful assessment of the family and social environment will help determine what interventions are needed.

Adherence

There is considerable evidence that persons with chronic illnesses do not follow through on the treatment regimens and protocols prescribed by health care professionals (Haynes, Taylor, & Sackett, 1979). This nonadherence may have disastrous results, including cessation of a presumed "unsuccessful" treatment, a decline in functioning, and damage to the patient–provider relationship in the form of guilt by the patient and anger by the provider. One of the many adaptations required by patients with arthritis is to incorporate a medical and personal disease management program into their lives. The term *adherence* is used here in preference to *compliance*, which is commonly found in nursing literature, because it is freer of the negative judgment implied in the labeling of a patient as *noncompliant*. Adherence recognizes the voluntary nature of the patient's participation in the medical regimen and implies a working partnership with the providers.

The chronic nature of rheumatic disease treatment regimens fosters poor adherence. The treatment regimens are complex, require daily effort, and may be somewhat uncomfortable. The results obtained from treatment are often slow in coming or may consist of preventing loss of function, which is not as reinforcing as the cessation of a painful condition. Other factors that have been linked to poor adherence include psychiatric illness, high anxiety, poor social support, and the need to carry out self-management skills alone. If the location of the treatment is inconvenient, or if the provider changes frequently or is viewed as unknowledgeàble, adherence is also likely to be poor. The community health nurse is often in the position of trying to implement a complex disease management program with a patient who has limited resources and is expecting a cure.

The patient must be assisted to assume responsibility for the management of the disease. Many patients, who have lived through the development of antibiotics and the subsequent conquest of most infectious diseases, simply cannot believe that medical science cannot cure their arthritis. They feel that it is the health care professional's responsibility to cure the disease. "If they cannot help me, what can I do?" is a frequently voiced question. Self-care for disease management becomes a difficult concept to accept. Patients naturally assume that if a cure is not possible, nothing can be done. They may abdicate responsibility for their treatment and care to the medical system and/or their family. The suffering due to their arthritis may then be compounded by the guilt they experience for burdening their family. The diagnosis or prevention of adherence problems and the development of self-management skills are effective antidotes.

Not every intervention strategy is appropriate for every patient. The nurse begins with the basic strategies that have been previously outlined. If these are insufficient, then strategies that are appropriate for the patient, nurse, and available resources must be developed. Some examples of strategies to cope with poor adherence and failure to take responsibility are listed in Table 7-8.

The strategies outlined in this table may be used to increase the patient's likelihood of following any medical recommendation. Problems with medication regimens, participation in ROM exercises, or the use of assistive devices may be the target of the intervention. All of these strategies require that additional time be spent with the patient, and some require the use of simple behavior modification

Table 7–8   Sample Strategies for Patients with Problems Related to Adherence

Establish a good relationship
Agree on goals and ways to reach them
 Use written commitments and contracts
Make cooperation easy
Teach the patient and family
Simplify the treatment regimen where possible
Reduce barriers to compliance where possible
 Cost, ease of access, time, complexity
 Use a problem-solving approach; develop alternatives
Build the changes into the patient's routine
Use compliance reminders: telephone calls, post cards, calendars
Develop a reinforcement program
 Reinforce cooperation
Provide increased supervision
 Increased home visits, rehospitalization if needed
Treat emotional problems that interfere
 Refer patient for additional help

principles. A general rule is to focus on only one or two new activities at a time. Once the patient has successfully mastered and accepted these activities, it will be easier to add new self-care skills in the future. It is extremely difficult for anyone to have to adopt an entirely new lifestyle with numerous required self-care behaviors. If the nurse starts with changes that are relevant to the patient's most important goals, she will have the greatest likelihood of success. Change will take time, and the process can usually not be hurried.

Unproven Treatments

The use of unproven treatments is related to limitations in insight. The scope of this problem in arthritis care was discussed in Chapter 1. The number of potential unproven treatments and remedies is limitless, restricted only by the bounds of the imagination. The Arthritis Foundation estimates that the vast majority of individuals with arthritis, perhaps as many as 90%, will experiment with or employ an unproven treatment at some point in their disease process (Kushner, 1984). Millions of dollars may be spent annually on drugs, diets, and devices that have never been scientifically tested.

The nature of the disease process of many types of arthritis, with the lack of cure, makes these patients particularly vulnerable to the inducements of unproven remedies. As discussed earlier in this chapter, the pattern of exacerbation and remission constantly interferes with the patient's ability to achieve and maintain control over the disease. During exacerbations, patients become vulnerable to advertising that promises cure and relief of pain. At the best of times, the arthritis regimen is both complex and time-consuming. New remedies are frequently introduced to patients by well-meaning family members and friends who correctly perceive that the patient wants help. It is difficult to criticize patients who are grasping at unproven remedies in their search for relief.

The primary concerns of the nurse are to educate the patient and family to evaluate advertising claims carefully, and to prevent physical harm as well as potential financial drain. The claims of unproven remedies are difficult to evaluate, as they frequently take the form of testimonials from individuals. In rheumatoid arthritis the disease pattern of exacerbation and remission makes it impossible to dismiss all such claims summarily. Science does not have all the answers when it comes to the individual's response to arthritis. The well-studied placebo effect further confuses the issue. The fact is that some patients do show a positive response to some unproven remedies. In these situations, the nurse's major concern is to ensure the patient's safety.

Dealing with the use of unproven treatments requires great skill and sensitivity on the part of the nurse. Considering the statistics, the nurse should probably assume that most patients have tried or will try such treatments at some time. Open communication and a good nurse–patient relationship are essential to any intervention in this area. The nurse must be sensitive to the patient's feelings and take care to avoid making the patient feel foolish or ignorant.

The assessment focuses on exploring what methods the patient uses or has used, including over-the-counter medications, vitamins, diets, lotions, exercises, machinery, equipment, and treatments. Besides eliciting data about what treatment methods have been used, the nurse attempts to uncover the reason behind their use, for that will be the focus of intervention. Countering the use of unproven methods with facts and rationales is rarely successful and may only result in breaking down the nurse–patient relationship. The proposed remedies should be evaluated for safety. If they are potentially harmful, the nurse must intervene and attempt to influence the patient to discontinue their use. Otherwise, patient autonomy should be respected as long as the treatment is used along with and not in place of the prescribed treatment regimen.

Unproven methods are an uncomfortable subject for health care professionals and raise concerns about patients being victimized. Therefore it is also appropriate for nurses to assist patients to develop their critical thinking skills. Nurses should be alert to media advertising about arthritis treatments and claims for cure, and should maintain files of examples. These can be used for educational purposes, assisting patients to analyze product or treatment claims critically. Table 7-9 outlines some cues that can be taught to patients to help them evaluate the claims of unproven treatments. Table 7-10 summarizes basic interventions in the area of limitations in insight in a care plan format.

The psychological and behavioral difficulties that may be encountered by patients adapting to chronic arthritis are many and varied. Most patients and families make the required adjustments well. The emphasis on adaptive alterations in psychological and behavioral areas in this chapter may lead the nurse to expect these difficulties to

Table 7–9   Recognizing Unproven Treatments: Cues That Indicate Unproven Remedies

1. A cure is offered or promised.
2. Testimonials and case histories are used as proof of the treatment's effectiveness.
3. The treatment is described as secret or exclusive.
4. The treatment is advertised only in sensational papers and magazines or through the mail.
5. Conventional treatment is condemned.
6. "Natural" methods, or nutrition remedies are claimed as cures.
7. Government agencies and the medical profession are accused of blocking progress by not approving the method.

Source: The Arthritis Foundation, excerpted from *Understanding Arthritis*. Copyright © 1984 Arthritis Foundation. Reprinted with the permission of Charles Scribners Sons, an imprint of Macmillan Publishing Company.

appear in every person, but this is *not* the case. The extensive, detailed description of these difficulties is provided to educate the nurse about what to be alert for, not what to expect. Treatment may be indicated in some cases, and prevention strategies are indicated in all cases. Many of the strategies outlined in this chapter can be used in a preventive as well as a therapeutic manner. The community health nurse is in a unique position to gather information and provide appropriate intervention and referral. Nursing intervention can be a crucial element in assisting patients to achieve the goal of effective self-management.

CASE STUDIES

1. Mrs. Susan Joseph is a 55-year-old widow with progressive rheumatoid arthritis. Her husband, on whom she had been extremely dependent, died suddenly last year. She went to live with her daughter immediately after her husband's death and has never returned to her own home. She has been depressed since her husband's death, and her recent disease exacerbations have significantly worsened her depression. She is passive and apathetic, showing little interest in her appearance or other aspects of her arthritis regimen. She does not follow her exercise prescription and simply lies in bed on bad days.

   Her daughter is both frustrated and upset. She loves her mother and is willing to have her live permanently with their family, but her helpless, apathetic behavior is wearing everyone down. She knows little about her mother's prescribed regimen and is unclear about how much and in what ways to direct her.

Table 7–10 Care Plan for Patients Experiencing Limitations in Insight

Nursing Diagnosis	Patient Goal	Nursing Intervention
Noncompliance[a] related to the complexity of the treatment regimen.	Patient actively participates in treatment regimen. Patient can verbalize and demonstrate components of treatment regimen. Patient will express commitment to goal set for treatment.	1. Provide patient education as indicated. 2. Encourage patient to express feelings about prescribed regimen. 3. Contract with patient as appropriate for essential behaviors. 4. Teach family to reinforce positive behaviors. 5. Insure that all decision making is collaborative. 6. Simplify regimen where appropriate.
Knowledge deficit related to unproven treatments.	Patient will verbalize how to identify an unproven treatment method. Patient will set goals and priorities within the total regimen.	1. Establish and maintain a trusting relationship with patient. 2. Explore patient's use of unproven methods. 3. Avoid judgmental interventions. 4. Assess for learning readiness. 5. Instruct patient in evaluation process for unproven treatment. 6. Reinforce involvement with prescribed treatment regimen.

[a]The term *noncompliance* is included in the care plan because it is the currently accepted North American Nursing Diagnosis Association nursing diagnosis for this problem.

1. What psychological or behavioral problems are evident in this situation? How might they be related to Mrs. Joseph's arthritis?

2. What goals will you try to establish with Mrs. Joseph?

3. What specific strategies will you employ to attempt to meet these goals?

4. What guidance should be offered to Mrs. Joseph's daughter? What teaching does she need to be helpful in this situation?

2. Patty Rogers is a 36-year-old woman with rheumatoid arthritis that was diagnosed 18 months ago. The disease exhibited a severe, rapid onset and thus far has responded poorly to all efforts at treatment control.

Ms. Rogers works as an administrative assistant and loves her work. She is concerned and anxious that she may have to quit her job, since her hand involvement is already extensive. Because she has always prided herself on her independence and self-reliance, this loss of control has unsettled her. She finds her reddened, swollen joints extremely unattractive, although she has never considered herself a vain person.

She arrives at the clinic anxious and angry. She questions the staff's competence and wonders why she should follow any of their guidelines when obviously "nothing works." "I may as well start trying some of these other ideas my family keep sending me," she concludes.

1. What behavioral problems are present in this situation? How might they be related to her arthritis?

2. What strengths does Ms. Rogers bring to this situation? What weaknesses?

3. What goals might be appropriate for Ms. Rogers?

4. What specific strategies might you employ to assist Ms. Rogers to meet these goals?

PATIENT EDUCATION MATERIALS

Arthritis Foundation. (1983). *Overcoming rheumatoid arthritis: What you can do for yourself.* Arthritis Foundation, 1314 Spring St., N.W., Atlanta, GA 30309.

Arthritis Foundation. (1983). *Taking charge: Learning to live with arthritis.* Arthritis Foundation, 1314 Spring St., N.W., Atlanta, GA 30309.

Hanson, I. (1980). *Outwitting arthritis.* Creative Arts Book Co., 833 Bancroft Way, Berkeley, CA 94710.

Missouri University. (1980). *Coping with arthritis.* University of Missouri,

Multipurpose Arthritis Center, Health Sciences Center, 807 Stadium Rd., Columbia, MO 65212.

National Institutes of Health. (1981). *How to cope with arthritis.* National Institute of Arthritis, Diabetes, Digestive and Kidney Disease, NIH Building 31, Room 9A04, Bethesda, MD 20205.

AUDIOVISUAL MATERIALS

Arthritis Foundation. (1978). *Arthritis quackery.* Arthritis Foundation, 1314 Spring St., N.W., Atlanta, GA 30309.

Dartmouth-Hitchcock Medical Center. (No date). *Living with arthritis.* Dartmouth-Hitchcock Arthritis Center, Dartmouth Medical Center, Hanover, NH 03756.

BIBLIOGRAPHY

Achterberg-Lawlis, J. (1982). The psychological dimensions of arthritis. *Journal of Consulting and Clinical Psychology, 50*(6), 984–992.

American Hospital Association (1982). *Strategies to promote self-management in chronic disease.* Chicago: AHA/CDC Health Education Project, Center for Health Promotion, American Hospital Association.

Anderson, R. O., Bradley, L. A., Young, L. D., McDaniel, C. K., & Wise, C. M. (1985). Rheumatoid arthritis: Review of psychological factors related to etiology, effects and treatment. *Psychological Bulletin, 98,* 358–387.

Becker, M. H., & Maiman, L. A. (1980). Strategies for enhancing patient compliance. *Journal of Community Health, 6,* 113–135.

Bradley, L. A. (1985). Psychological aspects of arthritis. *Bulletin on the Rheumatic Diseases, 35*(4), 1–12.

Brown, J. H., Spitz, P. W., & Fries, J. F. (1980). Unorthodox treatments in rheumatoid arthritis (abstract). *Arthritis and Rheumatism* (supplement), *23,* S657–658.

Burns, D. (1980). *Feeling good.* New York: William Morrow.

Cassileth, B. R., Lusk, E. J., Strouse, T. B., Miller, D. S., Brown, C. C., Cross, P. A., & Tenaglia, A. N. (1984). Psychosocial status in chronic illness: A comparative analysis of six diagnostic groups. *New England Journal of Medicine, 311,* 506–511.

Ferguson, J., & Bole, G. G. (1979). Family support, health beliefs and therapeutic compliance in patients with rheumatoid arthritis. *Patient Counseling and Health Education, 1*(3), 101–105.

Garber, J., & Seligman, M. E. P. (1980). *Human helplessness: Theory and application.* New York: Academic Press.

Hawley, D. (1984). Nontraditional treatments of arthritis. In D. Hawly (ed.), *Arthritis: Impact on people* (pp. 210–256). Philadelphia: W. B. Saunders.

Haynes, R. B., Taylor, D. W., & Sackett, D. L. (1979). *Compliance in health care.* Baltimore: Johns Hopkins University Press.

Higham, C., & Jayson, M. V. (1982). Nonprescribed treatments in rheumatic patients (abstract). *Annals of Rheumatic Disease, 41,* 203.

Kushner, I. (1984). *Understanding arthritis.* New York: Scribner's.

Miller, J. F. (1983). *Coping with chronic illness: Overcoming powerlessness.* Philadelphia: F. A. Davis.

Pigg, J. S., Driscoll, P. W., & Caniff, R. (1985). *Rheumatology nursing: A problem-oriented approach.* New York: Wiley.

Pitzele, S. K. (1985). *We are not alone: Learning to live with chronic illness.* Minneapolis: Thompson.

Rosenbaum, M. (1983). Learned resourcefulness as a behavioral repertoire for the self-regulation of internal events: Issues and speculations. In M. Rosenbaum, C. M. Franks, and Y. Jaffe (eds.), *Perspectives on behavioral therapy in the eighties* (pp. 54–73). New York: Springer.

Strategies to promote self-management in chronic disease. (1982). Chicago: AHA/CDC Health Education Project, Center for Health Promotion, American Hospital Association.

Zeibell, B. (1981). *Wellness: An arthritis reality.* Dubuque, Iowa: Kendall-Hunt.

PART 5

PHYSICAL ALTERATIONS

PHYSICAL ALTERATIONS

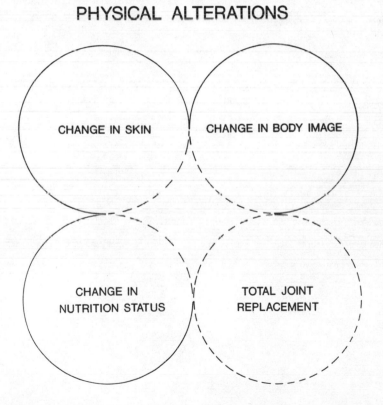

8

Physical Alterations After Total Joint Replacement

Trina Vecchiolla
Judith K. Sands

The basic treatment protocol for arthritis is composed of an appropriate balance of rest, exercise, medication, joint protection, and pain relief strategies, as discussed throughout this book. And, in most cases, arthritis can be successfully managed with this multifaceted treatment plan. However, in some cases, the joint damage of arthritis is so extensive that the standard treatment regimen is ineffective. Surgical intervention is then considered. Surgery has always played a role in arthritis management, but until quite recently that role was basically limited to repairing tendons and ligaments and fusing unstable joints. The development and refinement of total joint replacement procedures over the last several decades have produced dramatic changes in the role of surgery in arthritis management. Surgery is being used with increasing frequency in situations in which joint damage and chronic pain severely compromise an individual's ability to function. A significant number of arthritis patients have now been treated with total joint replacement, and the procedures have consistently been shown to successfully relieve pain, correct deformity, and improve both mobility and functional capabilities.

As surgical intervention in arthritis is used with increasing frequency, it is extremely likely that the community health nurse will be involved in the home care of arthritis patients after total joint replacement. Hospital stays for total joint replacement used to average several weeks, but the emphasis on hospital cost containment in the 1980s has steadily decreased the hospitalization period to the point where patients without complications can be discharged within 7–10 days. Discharge represents the beginning of recovery and rehabilitation after total joint replacement, however, not the end. Even strict Medicare reimbursement guidelines recognize the importance of home follow-up after total joint replacement and authorize it, along with needed physical therapy. The outlines of the rehabilitation regimen will have been carefully established during hospitalization, but success or failure is often at least partially dependent on the patient's own adherence to the regimen at home. The community health nurse can play a vital role in this process. It is therefore important that she understand the nature of the surgical procedures and the applicable nursing concerns during the postoperative and rehabilitation periods.

It is essential that patients who elect total joint replacement surgery do so with a complete and careful understanding of what is involved. The surgery itself represents the beginning of a rehabilitation process that may consume many months. The patient must understand that although relief of arthritis pain is a consistent outcome of this surgery, improvement of motion and function in the joint is much less predictable. The days and weeks of the home exercise and rehabilitation regimen may prove to be quite discouraging to the patient when the multidisciplinary supports of the inpatient hospital setting are removed. It is difficult, if not impossible, to predict in advance how any particular patient will respond to the surgery. However, patients with single-joint disease who are in basically good health often make remarkably fast recoveries. Patients with multiple joint involvement who are debilitated due to the overall effects of their disease, however, may face a protracted period of slow rehabilitation. All of these factors need to be understood and considered in making the decision to pursue surgical intervention. Whether the recovery is fast or slow, however, the community health nurse can play an important part in the rehabilitation process by knowledgeably supervising the home regimen and providing much needed support and encouragement along the way.

TYPES OF JOINT SURGERY

Total joint replacements are the best-known surgical procedures, but they are not the only type of surgical intervention used in arthritis. Table 8-1 briefly describes other types of surgical procedures that may be employed to deal with specific problems. Alternatives to joint replacements are often considered for younger patients who face uncertain disease activity in the future and for osteoarthritis patients whose joint disease may be more limited. Total joint replacements are the procedures of choice in most situations in which pain is the primary problem because their success in decreasing or eliminating joint pain has been particularly high.

Arthroplastic procedures in which new joints are surgically created have contributed the most exciting progress to arthritis care. Joint replacement surgery has been performed for over 25 years, but all of these procedures are still evolving, with changes in techniques and prosthetic components occurring frequently. The surgical outcomes are increasingly both successful and durable. Hopefully, progress will continue to be made as demands for the surgery escalate with an aging population.

To date, the hip and knee joints have been the principal targets of arthroplastic surgery, and the care involved in these procedures will be the focus of this chapter. These joints are not, however, the only ones for which surgery is employed.

Table 8–1 Joint Surgery Used in Arthritis

Type	Description	Uses
Arthroscopy	The use of a periscope instrument to visualize a joint directly for diagnosis or to perform surgery.	Diagnosing and assessing joint damage and/or removing or repairing cartilage damage.
Synovectomy	The removal of part or all of a joint's diseased synovium.	Primarily used to prevent excessive damage to and erosion of tendons and ligaments.
Osteotomy	Cutting and setting a bone in proper alignment.	To correct joint deformity and improve alignment.
Athrodesis	Fusion of the bones of a joint so that the joint is frozen and not movable.	To improve joint stability so that the joint may support weight bearing without pain.
Resection	The removal of all or part of a bone.	To correct deformities or remove painful bunions and improve weight bearing by reducing pain.
Arthroplasty	The rebuilding, relining, or replacement of damaged joints.	To reduce pain, correct deformity, and improve joint function.

The functions of the hand joints are particularly intricate. Arthritis frequently attacks these joints and causes serious functional losses, as well as some of the most common arthritis deformities. Surgery involving hand joints is usually aimed at improving function, reducing pain, and correcting deformities. Portions of the finger joints may be replaced with prostheses of a silicone rubber compound to correct deformities. Silastic hinges may be inserted to produce functional and cosmetic improvements, especially in the proximal joints. Arthrodesis, where a joint is surgically ankylosed and immobilized, may be used in the wrist to provide stability and reduce pain. The resulting loss of function can be compensated for to a remarkable degree. Total joint replacement is not commonly used for the wrist at this time due to the need for significant joint strength and tolerance for lifting.

Total joint replacement may be used in the shoulder joint when advanced disease is present, but it is not a common practice. The surgery is quite difficult technically and entails a protracted period of rehabilitation. In addition, the surgical outcome still allows for only limited shoulder movement. It does, however, eliminate the problem of unrelenting pain.

Pain and deformity resulting from arthritis in the feet can severely limit an individual's mobility, as these joints bear all of the body's weight. Multiple surgical procedures may be attempted in advanced disease. Arthrodesis of the bones of the ankle or at the back of the foot may increase stability. Bones in the arch of the foot or in the toes may be resected or replaced to correct deformities and improve mobility. Research is proceeding on a replacement prosthesis for the ankle joint.

Synovectomy, the removal of the synovial membrane and joint resurfacing are two surgical procedures that may be employed to reduce pain and improve function in the elbow joint. Total elbow replacement is available but is not yet as successful as total joint replacement in the hip or knee. The elbow joint lacks a significant covering of muscle and tissue to cushion the prosthesis adequately, and skin breakdown over the prosthesis is often an ongoing problem. Persistent dislocation of the elbow prosthesis remains another unsolved problem. Both of these problems should prove gradually amenable to ongoing research and prosthesis development.

It is important to reemphasize that while surgery is only part of a total arthritis treatment program, it can be a very important part, and it may lead to significantly improved mobility and general improvement in the patient's functional abilities. The remainder of this chapter will focus on the two most common forms of joint surgery—total joint replacement of the hip and knee. The major aspects of rehabilitation nursing care will be discussed through the role of the community health nurse in assisting patients to make a successful recovery.

TOTAL HIP REPLACEMENT

The hip was the first joint for which total joint replacement was attempted. Early and largely unsuccessful efforts date back to the 1920s and 1930s. Total hip replacement first became successful in the 1950s and 1960s, when low-friction prosthetic materials and long-lasting acrylic cements were developed. Since that time, the procedure has achieved widespread acceptance. Tens of thousands of Americans undergo total hip replacement annually, with excellent overall success rates. At least part of the success of total hip replacement can be attributed to the fact that most patients experience only manageable pain postoperatively and achieve significant functional improvement even if they do not adhere closely to the postsurgical rehabilitation and exercise plan.

Total hip replacement is used successfully with both rheumatoid arthritis and osteoarthritis. The surgery offers dramatic improvement to many individuals whose joint disease is so extensive that virtually constant pain, plus difficulty in walking and sitting, are daily realities. In its early phase, total hip replacement surgery was used only with older adults because of serious concerns about the durability and longevity of the prosthesis. Prosthesis loosening over

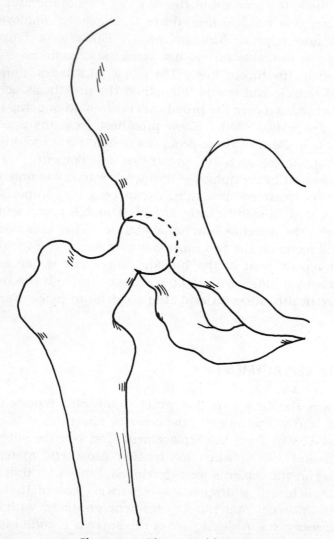

Figure 8–1. The normal hip joint.

time, largely the result of cement failure, is still a concern with joint replacement, but refinements in parts and techniques have raised the projected longevity of cemented joint prostheses to an average of 10–20 years. Preliminary data on the newer noncemented prostheses indicate an even longer projected life span. Total hip replacement is therefore being used increasingly in younger individuals whose disease has not yet become disabling.

Numerous types of procedures and prostheses are available today. Figures 8-1 and 8-2 illustrate the normal hip joint and a typical hip prosthesis. Metal, plastic, and ceramic parts are all used. Decisions

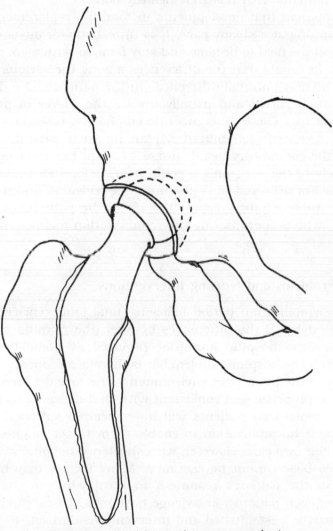

Figure 8–2. Total hip replacement prosthesis.

about which prosthesis to use are based on the patient's age and overall physical condition and on a careful assessment of the condition of the bone. The most common prostheses in current use are those with a femoral piece made of titanium and an acetabular piece made of silastic. These parts are usually held in place with a special bone cement, methylmethacrylate. Current research is focused on the use of prosthetic pieces with porous overlays that attempt to stimulate bony growth and a fusion between the bone and the prosthesis, thereby achieving a longer-lasting connection. Other cementless prostheses are also being researched for use, particularly with younger patients with relatively healthy bone.

It is apparent that developments in total hip replacement surgery are continuing at a steady pace. It is unrealistic for anyone not specializing in the field to become and stay familiar with all of them. It is therefore fortunate that the differences among the various surgeries necessitate only minimal differences in the patient's care during the rehabilitation period and usually involve the degree of permissible weight bearing. These differences do emphasize, however, the importance of a written rehabilitation plan for each patient. This plan enables the community health nurse to adapt her interventions appropriately to the surgeon's specific plan. Before adequate care can be planned or delivered, this plan must be reviewed, and it is critical that the nurse obtain a copy either from the patient, the physical therapist who is coordinating the rehabilitation regimen, or the surgeon.

Patient Problems and Nursing Interventions

As the hospitalization period following total joint replacement continues to shorten, the differences between the nursing care implemented in the hospital and that required at home become less significant. The hospital problem list is therefore adapted to meet the demands of the home care environment. The care delivered at home must be appropriate and consistent with that delivered in the hospital. It is hoped that patients will have received sufficient teaching during their hospitalization to enable them to act as effective partners in their own care. However, with shortened hospitalizations, this knowledge base cannot be assumed. Many factors may have interfered with the patient's readiness to learn while in the hospital. Therefore, each patient's knowledge base must be carefully assessed before goals are established and interventions devised.

Mobility and Exercise

The nursing diagnosis of impairment of mobility remains a significant concern in several areas during the rehabilitation period. The importance of proper positioning of the operative leg to prevent prosthesis dislocation is carefully taught to the postoperative patient and then demonstrated by the nurse. Throughout the hospitalization period, hip abduction will have been ensured by the continuous use of abduction splints or pillows. The patient is assisted in turning with the operative leg maintained in abduction. Positioning precautions must be continued during the early weeks after discharge. The greatest risk for prosthesis dislocation exists during the first 6 weeks after surgery and decreases with time as the muscles surrounding the new prosthesis regain strength and tone. Patients who have accepted the fact that positioning is extremely important may be quite fearful of sleeping in their own bed without special equipment or nurses available to assist with turning. Discharge teaching should therefore be reviewed, and patients should be reassured about the basic stability of the new hip. Several simple precautions should be carefully followed, however, to avoid adduction. Patients should not sleep on their operative side or turn to their unaffected side without a large bed pillow between the knees to prevent adduction and possible dislocation. They should not cross their legs, a movement that also causes acute hip adduction. Most patients would not consider crossing their legs while seated but might not realize that crossing their legs while lying in bed causes similar hip movement. Internal or external rotation of the leg while lying in bed should also be avoided for the same reason.

Avoiding excessive flexion of the hip is another mobility concern that carries over to the home setting, as acute hip flexion can also trigger prosthesis dislocation. A raised toilet seat should be in place for the patient's use, as low toilet seats are a common cause of excessive flexion. The same precautions apply to the use of low or deep chairs or sofas that force the hip into acute flexion. Pillows or cushions may be placed on soft furniture to decrease the flexion angle and thereby reduce the risk. During the first days at home, the sitting time in any chair should be limited to no more than an hour at a time. This restriction should also be carefully observed when sitting in an automobile. The nurse can assist the family to assess the home environment for furniture that the patient should either use or avoid. If possible, patients should use chairs with arms to facilitate proper rising and sitting. Table 8-2 and Figure 8-3 review the proper proce-

Table 8–2   Rising from a Chair

1. If possible, sit in chairs with arms for adequate support when getting up.
2. Move to the front edge of the chair before attempting to rise.
3. Stretch your affected leg well in front of you.
4. Tuck your unaffected leg well under the chair.
5. Use your arms and unaffected leg to raise yourself to a standing position.
6. Don't lean forward to stand up; keep your back straight.

dure for rising from a sitting position while avoiding excessive hip flexion. Patients should be asked to demonstrate this technique for the nurse and should then receive additional instruction if needed. The nurse should also explore and discuss with patients other normal daily activities, such as putting on shoes and picking up objects from the floor, that may put the hip in acute flexion. These activities can thereby be anticipated and avoided. Clearly, patients will require some assistance during this early phase of home rehabilitation.

While positioning restrictions have an obvious effect on the patient's mobility, exercise and ambulation comprise the other dimen-

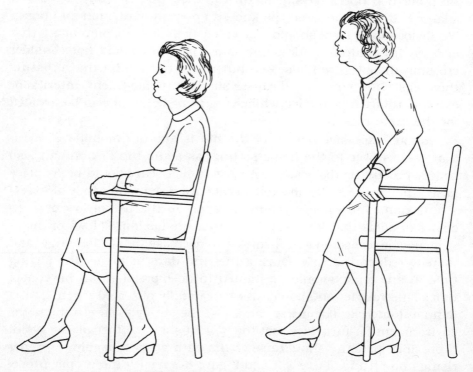

Figure 8–3. Rising from a chair.

sion of the diagnosis. Patients should be discharged with clear, specific written exercise plans. A call to the physical therapist or surgeon is indicated if a patient does not have this information, as there are many variations in exercise prescriptions. All patients should have received instructions on ankle, quadriceps set, and gluteal set exercises before surgery, as these exercises help to maintain adequate circulation and improve muscle tone for walking. Patients should be asked to demonstrate these exercises and should be offered further instruction if needed. Table 8-3 and Figures 8-4 and 8-5 review the basic steps of these exercises and can be used to assess the patient's understanding.

Most patients will use crutches or a walker as assistive devices for ambulation until full weight bearing is possible. Patients are usually discharged from the hospital with orders to "toe touch" only, which represents minimal weight bearing, or progressive weight bearing as tolerated. This crutch-walking gait is illustrated in Figure 8-6. The weight-bearing restrictions are set by the surgeon and usually reflect either the surgical approach used or the type of prosthesis inserted. Even patients who are initially restricted to toe touching will begin progressive weight bearing by about 6 weeks after surgery. Safe, ef-

Table 8–3   Exercises for Ambulation

Exercise	Technique
Ankle exercise	Alternately point the toes of the foot up and down, as in stepping on an automobile accelerator. This should be repeated 10–15 times at frequent intervals throughout the day.
Gluteal set*	Squeeze the buttocks muscles together and hold for a count of five before relaxing. Do at least 10 repetitions several times a day.
Quadriceps set*	Push the back of the knee down onto the bed while tightening the thigh muscle and hold for a count of five before relaxing. Repeat at least 10 times several times a day. Remember to exercise both legs.

*As with any isometric exercise, patients should rest for 10–20 seconds between contractions and should be cautioned not to hold their breath while tightening the muscle.

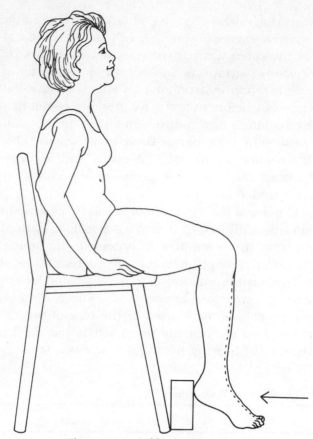

Figure 8–4. Ankle exercise.

fective crutch walking is essential during this early period. The home environment needs to be carefully assessed for hazards to crutch walking such as electrical wires, scatter rugs, and slippery floors. Patients should understand the importance of wearing supportive nonslip shoes when ambulating. They should also be able to state the symptoms of nerve pressure and damage that may be caused by the improper use of crutches. The nurse should ask patients to demonstrate their crutch-walking technique and reinforce the hospital teaching as needed. These concerns for patient safety are particularly important when a patient's home environment necessitates managing stairs. In climbing or descending stairs, the patient is instructed to always move the crutches with the affected leg. The affected leg is moved first when going downstairs and last when going up. Mastering stairs requires a significant amount of arm strength and can be

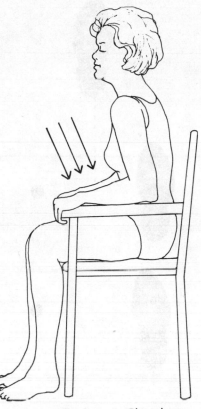

Figure 8–5. Gluteal set.

frightening for a patient who does not feel in control and balanced. Initially, it may be preferable to rearrange the patient's sleeping space, if this is feasible, or the patient may need to be referred for additional physical therapy teaching and supervised practice.

Patients will also have other prescribed exercises to practice during the rehabilitation period. The nurse needs to review these exercises with patients to ensure their understanding. Most of these exercises need to be continued for months after the surgery to foster optimal rehabilitation. The community health nurse can initiate care in this area by acknowledging how difficult it can be to persist in long-term exercise programs in the home. Together, then, the nurse and the patient can begin to explore obstacles to and facilitators of compliance. Patients may travel to a local hospital to receive physical therapy or have a physical therapist visit their home. It is crucial that the community health nurse assist patients to understand that these visits are an important aspect of the rehabilitation plan but are not

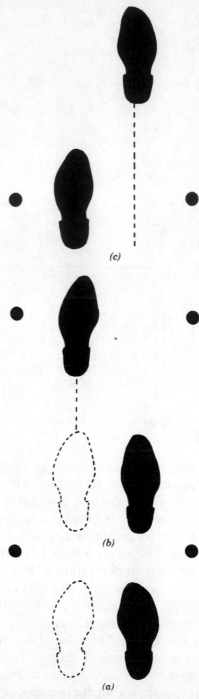

Figure 8–6. Three-point toe touch crutch gait. (a) tripod start position; (b) affected leg and both crutches are advanced together—weight is balanced on crutches; (c) unaffected leg is advanced.

Table 8–4   Precautions for Exercise

1. Use pain as your guide in moving the affected leg and avoid positions that cause pain.
2. Take frequent walks, but don't exhaust yourself.
3. Don't use your hand, strong leg, or anything else to force movement in your hip.
4. Don't allow anyone else to force movement in your leg. When exercising, let the leg move by itself.
5. Notify your physician immediately if you feel increased pain in your hip, or a sudden sharp pain or popping sound, or if you experience a loss of control over leg motion.

the *only* aspect. Patients must assume responsibility for continuing the exercise program on their own at home. Responsibility for self-care remains with the patient.

Even with a carefully followed exercise program, complications such as dislocation can arise. The nurse should review the signs and symptoms of complications and be sure that the patient has a written copy of the exercise precautions. These basic precautions are reviewed in Table 8-4.

Infection and Wound Healing

The potential for infection is the second major nursing diagnosis that carries over into the home rehabilitation period. Infection is one of the most dreaded complications of total hip replacement surgery. It is extremely difficult to treat effectively and may result in the need to remove the hip prosthesis. It may also entail weeks or even months of hospitalization. Every effort is made to protect the hip from infection during the hospitalization. The patient is thoroughly assessed for signs of concurrent infection before surgery. Patients are carefully assessed for the presence of asymptomatic urinary tract infection and may be referred for dental care before surgery is performed. The risk of migratory infection to the hip prosthesis is serious, particularly for patients who have received recent or ongoing steroid therapy. Meticulous skin preparation is performed, and prophylactic antibiotics may be given before surgery. Broad-spectrum antibiotics are routinely administered in the postoperative period, and the surgical incision is managed with frequent, thorough assessment and scrupulous aseptic technique for dressing changes.

Incision management carries over into the postdischarge period as patients are instructed to assess their healing incision regularly and to notify their surgeon if the hip becomes reddened or swollen or if a discharge from the incision is noted. The presence of fever or chills should also be reported. In addition, patients are usually instructed not to take tub baths or in any way to scrub the incision until healing is complete.

The concern about infection, however, is not limited to the healing of the surgical incision. Urinary tract infections are of particular concern, and patients must take active measures to prevent them. These infections are already a common problem among older adults, which makes prevention an even greater concern. If patients have no concurrent health problems that necessitate fluid restriction, they should be encouraged to increase their daily fluid intake significantly. Six glasses of water daily in addition to regular fluids is a good goal. Stasis of urine is one of the most common causes of urinary tract infection, and an adequate fluid intake is the best countermeasure. Frequent voiding to keep the bladder empty is another excellent intervention to prevent stasis. Patients should be encouraged to empty their bladders every 2–3 hours during the day. If patients have a history of infection, they may need to make dietary modifications in order to acidify the urine and thereby further inhibit bacterial growth.

All physicians involved in the patient's care should be informed of the hip prosthesis and be reminded of it before minor surgical procedures such as dental extractions. Prophylactic antibiotics are frequently administered before and after minor procedures to decrease the risk of migratory infection. This precaution needs to be continued indefinitely. Patients should also be instructed that the presence of a metal prosthesis can set off metal detector alarms in airports. Prior warning can avert a potentially embarrassing situation.

Sexuality

Sexuality is another area of concern during rehabilitation following total hip replacement. Painful arthritis involving the hip significantly affects the patient's ability to sustain sexual relationships with partners or spouses, but sexuality may not have been a concern verbalized during hospitalization. Sexuality concerns need to be assessed, and the nurse should not assume that patients have been counseled by their physicians. This is frequently not done. Sexual intercourse is usually prohibited during the first weeks at home, but intimacy can be gradually resumed if precautions are taken to avoid hip adduction and acute flexion. Arthritic hip pain can be both demoralizing and immobilizing. Relief from chronic pain may enable patients to enjoy sexual activity to a degree that was virtually impossible before hip replacement. Specific counseling concerning sexuality must be incorporated into the overall care plan. Chapter 4 deals in depth with concerns about sexuality in arthritis and offers approaches to both assessment and intervention.

Other concerns and patient problems may exist after total hip replacement to challenge home care management. Concurrent health problems produce special problems, as do environmental or social concerns existing in the home or the family. Patients with rheumatoid arthritis frequently have involvement of both hips and may face two replacement procedures with their subsequent restrictions, in a brief period of time. Regardless of the extent of the patient problems encountered, however, the basic nursing diagnoses discussed will always be a foundation for the home management care plan. These diagnoses and nursing interventions are summarized in Table 8-5 in a care plan format.

Table 8–5 Postdischarge Care Plan After Total Hip Replacement

Nursing Diagnosis	Patient Goal	Interventions
Impaired physical mobility related to: 1. Positioning and weight bearing restrictions.	Patient's hip surgery will heal without dislocation.	1. Maintain operative hip in abduction while in bed with bed pillows. 2. Use pillows between knees when turning in bed. 3. Do not cross legs while sitting or lying in bed. 4. Avoid acute hip flexion: Use a raised toilet seat. Avoid deep or low furniture or modify it as needed with pillows to prevent excessive flexion. 5. Follow correct steps when rising from a sitting position. 6. Avoid sitting for more than 1 hour at a time. 7. Use crutches or a walker as instructed by physical therapist. 8. Acquire assistive devices to avoid need for flexion during routine self-care activities.

continued

Table 8–5 Postdischarge Care Plan After Total Hip Replacement (*Cont.*)

Nursing Diagnosis	Patient Goal	Interventions
2. Discomfort and weakened muscle.	Patient will gradually regain full mobility in the affected hip and return to usual patterns of daily activity.	1. Continue to practice isometric exercises as instructed in the hospital. 2. Perform triceps exercises three times daily if using crutches to ambulate. 3. Assess home environment carefully for hazards to ambulation. 4. Reinforce exercise plan prescribed by physical therapist as needed. 5. Review signs and symptoms that indicate the development of complications.
Potential for injury related to infection of the surgical incision.	Patient's incision will heal without infection.	1. Maintain prescribed antibiotics for the full course of treatment. 2. Keep the incision dry and clean, free of all debris. 3. Assess the healing process daily. 4. Report any redness, swelling, or new discharge from the incision or the development of fever and chills. 5. Avoid tub baths until incision is completely healed. 6. Do not forcefully scrub the healing incision. 7. Report any onset of acute joint pain to physician immediately.
Knowledge deficit related to measures to employ in order to prevent complications in the hip.	Patient will employ measures to prevent the development of urinary tract infection.	1. Drink 6 glasses of water daily. 2. Avoid urinary stasis by emptying the bladder every 2–3 hours during the day. 3. Remain active and avoid immobility. 4. Check urinary pH once a week. Employ acid ash diet if urine is alkaline. 5. Inform all physicians of presence of hip prosthesis.

TOTAL KNEE REPLACEMENT

The knee joint is a relatively unstable joint that is subjected to heavy stresses throughout life. It is quite vulnerable to injury because of its relatively exposed position, and is also a common site for both degenerative and rheumatoid arthritis. Joint deterioration in the knee can cause significant problems with pain, posture, and ambulation. The refinement of effective fixative cements for total hip replacement procedures facilitated the development of prostheses for total knee replacement. The procedure's consistent success has made it extremely popular, and tens of thousands of total knee replacements are currently performed annually.

The development of satisfactory prostheses for total knee replacement has presented significant problems. Although the knee joint is classified as a hinge joint its structure and function are actually much more complex (see Figure 8-7). In addition to its hinge movement, the joint has a complex lateral rotary-type motion that is ex-

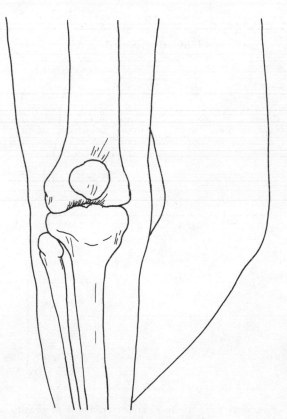

Figure 8—7. The knee joint.

tremely difficult to replicate in a prosthesis. Prostheses that function simply as hinges severely limit the overall mobility of the leg, especially during adjustments to inclines. Each new generation of prostheses has increased our ability to substitute artificial for normal joint movement. Figure 8-8a and b displays a commonly used knee prosthesis.

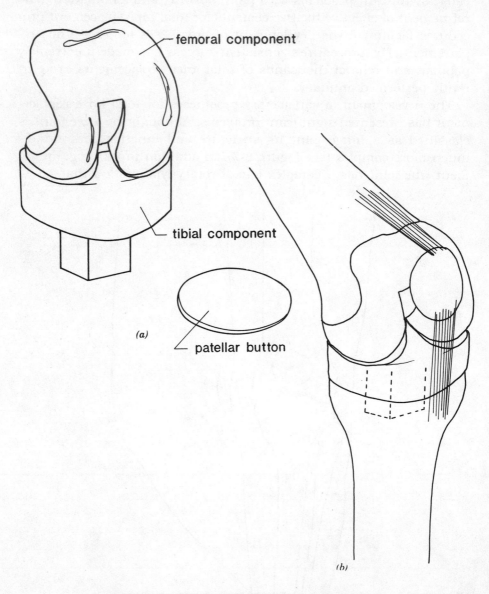

(a)

(b)

Figure 8–8. (a, b) Total knee replacement prosthesis.

Patient Problems and Nursing Interventions

The care considerations that carry over from the patient's hospitalization for total knee replacement to the home rehabilitation period share many features with the care described for total hip replacement patients. Impairment of mobility is, once again, a central nursing diagnosis with several subcomponents.

Mobility and Exercise

Positioning to prevent dislocation is less critical with a knee prosthesis than with a hip prosthesis because of the ease with which a knee immobilizer can be used to maintain the desired stability. Knee immobilizers control lateral movement in the knee joint and are generally used continuously, except when the patient is engaging in specific controlled exercise of the knee joint. The Zimmer knee splint or a hinged splint are among the most frequently used immobilizers. Regaining flexion capacity in the knee is a major goal of rehabilitation, but this is accomplished with a specific exercise regimen over time. About 180 degrees of knee flexion are required for walking without a limp, and this flexibility requires time and effort to achieve. Patients are again usually encouraged to avoid furniture and positions that require more than 90 degrees of flexion at the knee joint during their early weeks at home. A raised toilet seat is also suggested for comfort and safety. Restricting knee movement while encouraging patients to participate in a vigorous plan of knee exercises can create a confusing situation. It is important for patients to understand that casual and uncontrolled movement of the knee prosthesis during the early postoperative weeks can damage the new prosthesis and prevent effective healing.

Exercise and ambulation are the second major subcomponents of the diagnosis of impaired mobility. Most patients must use either a walker or crutches for initial ambulation after a total knee replacement. The degree of weight bearing permitted is again determined by the type of prosthesis implanted and the surgical technique employed, and these guidelines should be clearly stated by the surgeon or physical therapist in the written discharge instructions. A careful assessment of the patient's ability to use crutches or a walker safely in the home setting should be performed as discussed in the section on "Total Hip Replacement." The isometric exercises described in Table 8-3, which strengthen the muscles for ambulation, are again important for rehabilitation and should be reviewed with the patient. Whether or not patients are permitted to bear weight on the prosthesis, they will be encouraged to ambulate frequently throughout the day. Ambulation and exercise have the added benefit of supporting the peripheral circulation and helping to absorb the edema that tends to collect around the knee in the postoperative period. Edema is a common problem, as there is relatively little muscle tissue surrounding the knee joint and fluid reabsorption is fairly poor.

Although total knee replacement is an established and highly successful surgery, its outcomes are far less certain than those of total hip replacement and require a significant commitment on the part of the patient. It is hoped that these facts will have been carefully presented to the patient before surgery, but it is impossible to know how much teaching was absorbed or believed. Ongoing assessment of the patient's motivation, and ability to tolerate pain and participate in active rehabilitation, is essential.

Specific exercises will have been prescribed for the patient to help achieve a maximum amount of controlled knee flexion. This is a slow process that may be accompanied by a fair amount of discomfort. Some patients are treated in the postoperative period with continuous passive motion (CPM) devices, which attempt to accomplish earlier and more complete return of knee function while preventing phlebitis and hematoma formation. Because of the problems with adequate wound healing that seem to be asscoiated with the use of CPM machines, the appropriateness of their use is debated. Treatment with CPM machines is, however, an approved therapy under Medicare reimbursement guidelines, and the community health nurse may need to supervise patients who use these devices. The problem of achieving complete wound healing while simultaneously mobilizing the knee remains unsolved. When the patient is discharged, the nurse will need to review the prescribed exercise regimen and ask for a correct demonstration of the various flexion and straight leg-raising exercises. If a CPM machine has been prescribed, it is essential that the patient be visited immediately to ensure that the treatment plan can be safely and effectively implemented in the home environment. It is critical that the community health nurse reinforce with the patient the importance of the exercise regimen in the overall rehabilitation plan. The patient will need a great deal of emotional support in dealing with the ongoing discomfort and the sometimes slow nature of the progress. Whether the patient visits a physical therapy department as an outpatient or is visited at home by a physical therapist, these visits will constitute only a portion of the overall exercise time. Patients need to understand that the progress made from this point on is largely a matter of their own efforts and determination.

Infection and Wound Healing

The potential for infection is again of major importance during home rehabilitation following total knee replacement. Swelling of the knee and clear drainage from the incision may continue to be present during the rehabilitation period, especially after exercise. Patients must be taught to assess the incision daily for signs of inflammation and to evaluate any discharge carefully for a change in smell or appearance. The physician should be contacted if signs of infection develop or if fever or chills occur. Uncontrollable infection remains a serious concern with all joint replacement surgery, as it can result in failure of the prosthesis and loss of the joint itself. Therefore the patient should be taught to implement all of the other general precautions for preventing infection that are outlined in the discussion of total hip replacement. Table 8-6 summarizes in a care plan format the basic concerns of the rehabilitation period after total knee replacement.

Table 8–6 Postdischarge Care Plan After Total Knee Replacement

Nursing Diagnosis	Patient Goal	Interventions
Impaired physical mobility related to pain and weight-bearing restrictions	Patient will observe activity restrictions until incision is completely healed.	1. Use knee immobilizer at all times when not performing specific exercises. 2. Avoid acute knee flexion by: Using raised toilet seat. Avoiding use of low seats. 3. Use crutches or walker as instructed by physical therapist. 4. Use assistive devices as needed to maintain maximum independence during self-care.
	Patient will regain full flexion and extension range in knee.	1. Continue exercise program prescribed by physical therapist. 2. Provide support and encouragement. 3. Exercise regularly, using pain as a guide for extent.

continued

Table 8–6   Postdischarge Care Plan After Total Knee Replacement (*Cont.*)

Nursing Diagnosis	Patient Goal	Interventions
		4. Ambulate with crutches or walker frequently for short distances.
		5. Review signs and symptoms indicating problems with the prosthesis.
Potential impairment of skin integrity related to slow healing of surgical incision.	Patient's incision will heal without injury or infection.	1. Assess incision daily.
		2. Change dressings as indicated by presence of drainage.
		3. Report any redness, increased swelling, or change in the character of the drainage or the development of fever or chills.
		4. Do not soak or scrub healing incision.
		5. Seek prompt medical attention for infection occurring elsewhere in the body.

CASE STUDIES

1. Joe Beard is a 42-year-old man who has been experiencing steadily increasing pain and limitation of movement in his left hip. He developed degenerative osteoarthritis in the joint after suffering severe joint trauma in an automobile accident during his college years. He has compensated well up to the last 6 months, when increasing pain and stiffness significantly interfered with his ability to perform his job as a high school gym teacher. Joe is 6 feet 3 inches, weighs 200 pounds, and describes himself as being in excellent health except for his "bum hip."

   Joe's physician has recommended a total hip replacement, but Joe is extremely ambivalent and afraid of the surgery. He asks, "Don't you think I'm too young for an artificial hip? Isn't that what they do for old people who are really crippled from arthritis?" His wife is encouraging him to have the surgery, since the other alternative seems to be a classroom assignment teaching health and driver's education. She thinks that he will be miserable being so inactive. The Beards are comfortable financially, have adequate health insurance, and live in a roomy ranch house.

   1. How would you answer Joe's questions?

2. What are the advantages and disadvantages of total hip replacement in Joe's situation?

3. Is Joe a good candidate for surgery at this time? Why or why not?

4. What factors in his physical and social situation would be strengths or limitations if he decides to have the surgery?

5. After surgery, what assessments are essential to plan his home care? What care-planning factors do you consider to be most important?

2. Mrs. Sandra Taylor is a 63-year-old widow who has had rheumatoid arthritis for 25 years. Despite aggressive treatment, she has suffered frequent disease exacerbations and has gradually become disabled. She has had bilateral hip replacements in the last 5 years but still suffers from significantly restricted mobility as a result of increasing pain and dysfunction in both knees. Joint disease in her hands, wrists, and shoulders has left her with extremely limited muscle strength and endurance.

Mrs. Taylor is secure financially and has adequate health insurance coverage. She lives in a single-family split-level house with groups of six steps between the bedroom, living, and cooking areas. Mrs. Taylor has daily household help. Although she has no family, she has a wide network of friends who offer her ongoing companionship and assistance.

Mrs. Taylor's doctor recommends total replacement of both knees. Mrs. Taylor is very upset. She says, "I just don't think I can face all that pain again. I'm not very brave. I got so depressed after my last surgery."

1. Is Mrs. Taylor a good candidate for total knee replacement? Why or why not?

2. What factors in her physical and social situation would you consider as strengths? What factors are limitations?

3. If Mrs. Taylor has surgery, what assessment factors are essential to consider before home care is initiated? What assistance or assistive devices will she need?

4. What priorities would you set for her home care? What would be realistic goals? What nursing interventions might assist her to achieve them?

PATIENT EDUCATION MATERIALS

Arthritis Foundation. (1980). *Living with arthritis: A guide to total hip replacement.* Arthritis Foundation—Connecticut Chapter, Box 376, Withersfield, CT 06109.

Arthritis Foundation. (1982). *Surgery: Information to consider.* Arthritis Foundation—Patient Services Dept., Box 19000, Atlanta, GA 30326.

Carpenter, E. S. (1979). *Information for our patients about total knee joint replacement.* Professional Staff Association, Rancho Los Amigos Hospital, 7413 Golondinas St., Downey, CA 90242.

Cooke, D. (1984). *Surgery—a serious decision but often a beneficial one.* Arthritis Society, 920 Yonge St., Suite 420, Toronto, Ontario M4W 3J7, Canada.

Rheumatic Disease Program. (1980). *You and your new hip.* Columbia Hospital Rheumatic Disease Program, 2025 E. Newport Ave., Milwaukee, WI 53211.

AUDIOVISUAL MATERIALS

Arthritis Foundation. (1980). *Surgery.* Arthritis Foundation—New York Chapter, 115 E. 18th St., New York, NY 10003.

Thomas, L. A. (1982). *Your operation: Total hip replacement.* Encyclopedia Britannica Educational Corp., 425 N. Michigan Ave., Chicago, IL 60611

BIBLIOGRAPHY

Blaha, J. D., & Pickett, J. C. (1985). Controversy on total knee arthroplasty. *Clinical Orthopedics and Related Research, 192,* 2–112.

Burton, K. E., Wright, V., & Richards J. (1979). Patients' expectations in relation to outcome of total hip replacement surgery. *Annals of the Rheumatic Diseases, 38*(5), 471–474.

Doheny, M. O. (1985). Porous coated femoral prosthesis: Concepts and care considerations. *Orthopaedic Nursing, 4*(1), 43–45.

Levy, R. H. (1985). Progress in arthritis surgery: With special reference to current status of total joint arthroplasty. *Clinical Orthopedics and Related Research, 200,* 299–321.

Meyers, M. H., McNelly, D. B., & Nelson, K. (1978). Total hip replacement, a team effort. *American Journal of Nursing 28*(9), 1485–1489.

Roush, S. E. (1985). Patient perceived functional outcomes associated with elective hip and knee arthroplasties. *Physical Therapy, 65,* 1496–1502.

Spindler, C. E. (1984). Audiovisual preoperative teaching for the total hip patient. *Orthopaedic Nursing, 3,* 30–40.

Strang, E. L., & Johns, J. C. (1984). Nursing care of the patient treated with continuous passive motion following total knee arthroplasty. *Orthopaedic Nursing, 3*(6), 27–32.

Walsh, R., & Wirth, C. R. (1985). Total knee arthroplasty: Biomechanical and nursing considerations. *Orthopaedic Nursing*, 4(1), 29–34.

Wolfgang, G. (1984). Total hip arthroplasty: Picking the right candidate helps determine success. *Consultant*, 24, 211–222.

Wong, S., Wong, J., & Nolde, T. (1984). Total hip replacement: improving posthospital adjustment. *Nursing Management*, 15(4), 34A–34G.

9

Nutrition and Diet Therapy

Judith K. Sands

The role of nutrition and diet in the development and/or treatment of arthritis has intrigued both researchers and patients for over half a century. Diet therapy is one of the most commonly employed unproven treatments for arthritis and the source of much controversy in both lay and scientific literatures.

Although nutrition has been a topic of intense interest for many years, it has only recently been the subject of careful research. Most early diet studies were not carefully designed, and often grouped together individuals with diverse and varied forms of arthritis. Outpatient diet research is challenging and difficult under the best of circumstances, since rigorous control of the diet is almost impossible to achieve. Poor study designs, however, compounded the existing problems and produced results that were difficult to interpret and usually impossible to replicate.

Over the years, the Arthritis Foundation and most arthritis treatment centers have taken a very conservative approach to nutrition and simply advocate a sensible balanced diet. This approach is based on the fact that no diet has thus far been proven to cure arthritis or cause its symptoms to become either better or worse. This position, of course, excludes primary gout, with its well-documented relationship to levels of dietary purine. The large number of diets discussed in the literature is considered to be a fairly reliable indication that diet is not an effective treatment. Recent advances in our understanding of cellular nutritional processes, however, particularly in relation to the immune response, are causing researchers to consider that perhaps our knowledge concerning diet and arthritis is still incomplete. Nurses who work with arthritis patients must attempt to remain informed concerning nutritional research and assist patients to make sensible decisions concerning their personal diet and eating patterns.

NUTRITION AND ARTHRITIS

Individuals with arthritis often have abnormal serum levels of various dietary substances. The research challenge has been to attempt to determine whether these abnormalities are a result of the arthritis disease process or possibly one of its causes. Researchers have also attempted to determine whether correction of these nutritional imbalances has any effect on the patient's disease activity or clinical status. The nutritional elements that have been most thoroughly investigated are outlined below.

Zinc

The dietary element zinc has received a great deal of attention because serum zinc levels are typically low in persons with rheumatoid arthritis. Adequate amounts of zinc are important for proper wound and ulcer healing and for the maintenance of certain cellular immune responses. Zinc also appears to have limited anti-inflammatory effects. Oral zinc therapy has therefore been fairly thoroughly researched, but the results are inconclusive. In studies by Simkin (1981) and Job, Menkes, and Delbarre (1980), patients who were treated with oral zinc responded better than their placebo-treated counterparts, but the clinical improvements were neither statistically significant nor consistent. Zinc is therefore considered to be of potential benefit in the treatment of rheumatoid arthritis, but much more research is needed.

Copper

Copper is another dietary element that has received a lot of research attention. Persons with rheumatoid arthritis are consistently found to have higher serum levels of copper than the normal population. These levels can be as much as twice normal. Patients who are successfully treated with drugs such as penicillamine and experience an improvement in clinical function also usually experience a decrease in their serum copper level. However, dietary modification of the copper level has not produced any effect on the symptoms of rheumatoid arthritis or its clinical course. Researchers have therefore concluded that the serum copper elevation is a secondary effect of the systemic inflammation of rheumatoid arthritis and not a primary nutritional aberration influencing the disease process. Similar conclusions have also been drawn concerning frequently encountered variations in sulfur levels.

Iron

Mild to moderate anemia is a common finding in patients with rheumatoid arthritis. It is a hypochromic normocytic form of anemia that appears to be the result of a decreased use of endogenous iron in the body. It is therefore not a typical iron deficiency anemia. Although iron is available in the body, it is not incorporated properly into the red blood cells. This anemia is a challenging clinical feature of the disease because it is only marginally responsive to iron therapy. It can, however, contribute significantly to the patient's overall fatigue and activity intolerance. This iron disorder is thought to be an effect of chronic disease rather than a direct component of arthritis pathology. Correction or improvement of the clinical anemia can improve the patient's overall well-being, but it will not influence the disease or its symptoms.

Vitamins

Several vitamins have been investigated for their possible etiologic or therapeutic roles in arthritis. Vitamin C has received intense scrutiny, since it has been shown to possess some capacity to enhance the immune response. Levels of vitamin C are frequently low in patients with rheumatoid arthritis. Neither routine nor megadose supplementation of Vitamin C, however, has been shown to have any effect on the disease process. Similar results have also been found with vitamin B_6 (pyridoxine), which is also typically reduced in persons with rheumatoid arthritis. Treatment with vitamin E also cannot be proven to play any significant therapeutic role. At this point in our understanding of the treatment of arthritis, vitamin therapy has not been shown to alter the course of the disease.

Prostaglandins and Dietary Fatty and Amino Acids

A great deal of current basic research is focused on the production of prostaglandins and their apparently central role in the mediation of the body's immune response. Research in mice has shown that humoral immunity is impaired when there is a deficiency in fatty acids, and it is hypothesized that their levels could play a role in the course of rheumatoid arthritis. But since there are multiple fatty acids and many types of prostaglandins, a great deal of research will be needed to determine if their enhancing or suppressing effects on inflammation can be influenced by diet. While most of the data cannot yet be applied to actual treatment, they are both interesting and provocative. It is clear that nutritional research will focus increasingly on efforts to preserve and sustain immune competence.

Inflammation and Body Protein

As the general importance of body protein has become increasingly clear, attention has been focused on the effects of acute and chronic inflammation on the body's nutritional state. Any systemic metabolic insult that triggers the inflammatory response also produces a consistent metabolic and humoral response.

During the first few days, the metabolic response is in an acute phase characterized by hyperglycemia, hypoinsulinemia, glycogenolysis, and elevated free fatty acid levels. It next enters a chronic stage that persists as long as the inflammation is present. There is an ongoing release of endogenous corticosteroids that produces elevated glucose levels and rapid protein catabolism. Although the process is not nearly as devastating as the one that accompanies severe burns, it is similar in many ways. The individual's protein requirements are elevated, yet exogenous protein is used much less efficiently than usual. Normal metabolic balances are not reestablished until the inflammation is successfully controlled.

A negative nitrogen balance is no longer regarded as an undesirable but not terribly serious state. Its effects on wound and tissue healing have been well documented for years. Catabolic patients are immune deficient and may not respond appropriately to common antigens. Both morbidity and mortality rates are increased in hospitalized catabolic patients, especially the elderly. While a simple starvation state results primarily in the loss of adipose tissue, catabolism triggered by inflammation can cause up to 50% of the body's losses to occur from lean muscle tissue. This loss occurs regardless of the individual's body weight.

The implications for rheumatoid arthritis patients who experience disease exacerbations can be significant. Frequent or uncontrolled disease flare-ups can leave the person at substantial risk for other concurrent injuries or infections. The process also typically produces anorexia, which makes nutritional intervention more difficult. Aggressive nutritional therapy is felt to be indicated whenever protein malnutrition is suspected, especially as the condition may not be accompanied by a low body weight or a chronically malnourished appearance.

NUTRITION AND DIET ASSESSMENT

Despite the uncertainties concerning the role of nutrition in the causation and treatment of arthritis, the importance of an adequate nutritional status is unquestioned. Adequate assessment of an individual's nutritional status is an important foundation for counseling and intervention, and will require careful consideration of multiple objective and subjective factors.

Basic assessment begins with height and weight determinations and a general evaluation of their balance for the individual's frame size. These data can be compared with a standard height-weight guide such as that shown in Table 9-1. Information about the indi-

Table 9–1   Height and Weight Tables, Metropolitan Life Insurance Company, 1983

Height	Small Frame	Medium Frame	Large Frame
	Men		
5'2"	128–134	131–141	138–150
5'3"	130–136	133–143	140–153
5'4"	132–138	135–145	142–156
5'5"	134–140	137–148	144–160
5'6"	136–142	139–151	146–164
5'7"	138–145	142–154	149–168
5'8"	140–148	145–157	152–172
5'9"	142–151	148–160	155–176
5'10"	144–154	151–163	158–180
5'11"	146–157	154–166	161–184
6'0"	149–160	157–170	164–188
6'1"	152–164	160–174	168–192
6'2"	155–168	164–178	172–197
6'3"	158–172	167–182	176–202
6'4"	162–176	171–187	181–207
	Women		
4'10"	102–111	109–121	118–131
4'11"	103–113	111–123	120–134
5'0"	104–115	113–126	122–137
5'1"	106–118	115–129	125–140
5'2"	108–121	118–132	128–143
5'3"	111–124	121–135	131–147
5'4"	114–127	124–138	134–151
5'5"	117–130	127–141	137–155
5'6"	120–133	130–144	140–159
5'7"	123–136	133–147	143–163
5'8"	126–139	133–150	146–167
5'9"	129–142	139–153	149–170
5'10"	132–145	142–156	152–173
5'11"	135–148	145–159	155–176
6'0"	138–151	148–162	158–179

Source: Courtesy Statistical Bulletin, Metropolitan Life Insurance Company.

vidual's desired or ideal weight and body image should also be obtained.

Body weight can be an extremely important consideration in both rheumatoid and osteoarthritis. Many patients with osteoarthritis are overweight, which can place significant additional stress on their involved joints. Weight reduction may become a major focus for nursing intervention. Patients with rheumatoid arthritis tend to be normal in weight or underweight. Unplanned weight loss becomes an important assessment feature for these patients, as it may represent the catabolic stress response to chronic inflammation. Fatigue, anorexia, pain, and depression can also contribute to unplanned weight loss and should be carefully considered.

Most patients with arthritis consume daily diets that are adequate to meet their minimum daily requirements although a study of rheumatoid arthritis patients (Kowsari et al., 1983) found their diets to be at least marginally inadequate in some essential nutrients. Where the nutritional status is basically adequate, the assessment focus is on determining basic eating patterns and habits as a foundation for general nutrition counseling. The patient's food beliefs, general knowledge of nutrition, and use of vitamins, minerals, and other supplements is considered.

An additional focus for assessment will emerge if the nurse believes or suspects the patient to be nutritionally deficient. Persons at particular risk include the elderly, those who live alone and are responsible for their own shopping and cooking, those with limited financial resources, those with multiple joint involvement or significant self-care limitations, and those with frequent inflammatory exacerbations who may develop protein malnutrition from catabolism.

A simple dietary recall questionnaire is usually sufficient to provide a rough nutritional assessment even if the food intake is not broken down and analyzed for specific nutrient content. A 3-day food diary that can be left with the patient is usually adequate if combined with a simple recall questionnaire such as the one shown in Table 9-2. If completed as part of a nutrition interview, a simple tool such as this can provide considerable data about the patients basic diet pattern and balance.

Physical assessment findings can augment the data base with patients who are at true risk for malnutrition. Table 9-3 outlines some of the basic deviations from normal that could be indicative of a state of malnutrition. These specific symptoms may, of course, accompany other conditions, but their presence in a cluster is a fairly clear indication of a malnourished state. Sophisticated nutritional assess-

Table 9–2 Sample Diet Questionnaire

Please indicate which of the following foods you eat and how often.

Foods	Frequency		
	Hardly Ever	At Least Once a Week	Almost Everyday
Cheese, yogurt, ice cream	_____	_____	_____
Milk	_____	_____	_____
Meat—beef, pork, lamb	_____	_____	_____
Poultry—chicken and turkey	_____	_____	_____
Fish and shellfish	_____	_____	_____
Fruit and fruit juice	_____	_____	_____
Vegetables—raw or cooked	_____	_____	_____
Dried beans, peas, peanut butter	_____	_____	_____
Bread, cereal, tortillas	_____	_____	_____
Rice, pasta, grits, potatoes	_____	_____	_____

If you eat fruits or juices almost every day, which three do you eat most often? __
If you eat vegetables almost every day, which three do you eat most often? _____
How many meals do you usually eat each day? _____
Do you usually snack between meals? _____
If yes, what three snacks do you have most often? _____
Who shops for and cooks your meals? _____
Do you take supplemental vitamins or minerals? _____
If yes, what kind and how often? _____

Table 9–3 Physical Findings Indicative of Malnutrition

Body Area	Finding
Hair	Hair dull and dry, thin and sparse
Eyes	Pale conjunctivae, dryness of eye membranes, ring of fine blood vessels around cornea
Lips	Redness and swelling, cracking and fissures at corners of mouth
Tongue	Swelling, scarlet or purplish color
Gums	Recessed, spongy, and bleed easily
Nails	Spoon shaped, brittle, and ridged
Skin	Dryness, flaking, loss of fat
Muscles	Wasted, atrophic appearance

ment is rarely needed, although the nurse may need to refer patients to their physicians for appropriate blood tests. The serum albumin level is a fairly reliable reflection of protein intake and the degree of catabolic stress; a complete blood count and serum iron levels can help to establish the origins and severity of any clinical anemia; and an anergy panel where the individual's immunologic response to selected common antigens is measured may be used to provide a rough assessment of immune system competence.

NUTRITION AND DIET INTERVENTION

Since the importance of optimal nutrition in chronic illness is widely accepted, it is usually appropriate to establish a patient goal directed at improving nutritional status. The appropriate nursing interventions may vary significantly, however, from one patient situation to another.

Weight Control

Overweight is a chronic health problem among adults in the United States and is common in patients with osteoarthritis. There is little doubt that excess body weight increases the stress placed on weight-bearing joints such as the hip and knee. Overweight is also more difficult to reverse in persons with arthritis because the classic pain, stiffness, and fatigue may significantly limit the patient's ability to burn excess calories through increased physical activity.

Overweight can be simplistically described as the result of an overconsumption of calories in proportion to those burned as energy. The condition can be corrected by reducing total intake, increasing energy expenditure, or both. Anyone who has battled overweight, however, knows that the condition and its correction are far more complicated than this description indicates. Eating is a highly social experience in our society and is used for a wide variety of purposes in addition to providing basic nourishment. For many individuals, food is a basic and highly effective coping mechanism. The pain, mobility, and self-care limitations, sleep disturbances, depression, role and self-concept changes that may accompany arthritis can all be endured more easily by some patients by overeating.

Individuals are rarely unaware that they are overweight and rarely unaware of the negative consequences of obesity to their health. The nurse must establish the patients' feelings and goals about their excess weight before attempting to intervene in this sensitive area. If the individual is not ready to deal with the problem, preaching or teaching about the risks and evils of obesity will only serve to disrupt the nurse–patient relationship. If, however, patients desire to attempt to lose weight, the nurse can either assist them to develop a diet plan or refer them to an organized weight loss program or group.

If the needed weight loss is small or the patient's resources are strictly limited, an individualized home plan is probably desirable. The nurse explores both successful and unsuccessful diet efforts that the patient has used in the past. A simple food diary can be useful for assisting patients to become aware of the foods and quantities they eat. The patient and nurse can then work together to consider food preferences and priorities and ways in which calories can be reduced most painlessly. If patients are seriously overweight, they should be encouraged to join a formal weight loss group such as Weight Watchers. Weight loss is both stressful and frustrating, and most individuals profit from the support and encouragement of a peer group. Involvement of the family is always critical to a successful weight loss effort. It may be possible to involve another family member in the diet.

Exercise should be a part of every weight reduction program, but the use of active aerobic exercise may need to be restricted with arthritis patients. The nurse encourages patients to be as active as possible and teaches them that decreasing activity levels will necessarily require them to reduce their total caloric intake. Even normal-weight individuals need to be cautioned to monitor their weight carefully and to adjust their eating patterns gradually in response to decreasing activity.

Inadequate Nutrition

Inadequate nutrition presents the nurse with a different set of challenges. The patient may or may not be underweight, but experiences inadequate nutrition from the wrong mix or balance of foods or from inappropriate responses to the challenges of fever, inflammation, pain, anorexia, or fatigue.

The daily adult diet must include over 40 separate essential substances for good nutrition. Variety in the diet is essential, since no food provides all needed nutrients and many foods provide only a few. Despite the consistent appearance of diet or nutrition books on the best-seller lists, most individuals in our society are not well informed about the basics of good nutrition. The nurse cannot assume an adequate knowledge base about the basics of nutrition.

Basic Balanced Diet

Sound nutrition is built around regular ingestion of foods from the four basic food groups as outlined in Table 9-4. These basic recommendations are appropriate for all individuals with arthritis. In addition, however, the nurse should instruct the patient about the importance of including milk products in the daily diet as an important source of calcium. It is difficult to achieve adequate amounts of calcium in the diet without including dairy products. Skim milk products can be recommended when total calories must be controlled. Teaching about calcium is particularly important for postmenopausal women at high risk for osteoporosis.

Arthritis patients should also be encouraged to ensure that a regular portion of their bread and cereal exchanges is in the form of whole grains with natural fiber. Research findings point clearly to the central role of fiber in maintaining optimal bowel health.

Protein is abundant in the average American diet, but patients should be encouraged to reduce the quantity of red meat in their diet and increase their consumption of poultry and fish. American diets remain heavily skewed toward red meat ingestion despite the research that supports the importance of dietary changes for healthy

Table 9–4 Basic Daily Food Recommendations

Food Group	Servings	Serving Size
Milk	Two servings daily	1 cup (1 ounce cheese = 1 cup)
Vegetables and fruits	One vitamin A rich 　Dark green or deep yellow	½ cup
	One vitamin C rich 　Other raw vegetables 　Citrus and other fruits Two other vegetables or fruits	½ cup
Bread and cereal	Four servings daily 　Whole grains	1 slice bread ½–¾ cup pasta 1 ounce cereal
Protein	Two servings	2—3 ounces lean meat or poultry 2 eggs

Table 9–5   Essential Vitamins

Vitamin	Food Sources	Comment
	Water Soluble Vitamins	
Vitamin C (ascorbic acid)	Citrus fruit, berries, raw leafy vegetables	Minimal body storage, so needed daily.
Vitamin B_1 (thiamine)	Widely distributed in plant and animal foods, whole grains, green vegetables	Significant losses in high-temperature cooking.
Vitamin B_2 (riboflavin)	Milk, organ meats, eggs, breads and cereals	Destroyed by exposure to light.
Vitamin B_3 (niacin)	Proteins—organ meats, poultry, fish, whole grains	Stable in foods.
Vitamin B_6 (pyridoxine)	Meat, poultry, and fish, leafy vegetables, cereals	Need increases slightly with age.
Vitamin B_{12}	Animal foods	Some stored in liver. Heat destroys some of it.
	Fat-Soluble Vitamins	
Vitamin A	Liver, egg yolk, milk and cheese, dark green leafy vegetables, deep yellow fruits and vegetables	Stored in liver. Excess amounts can be toxic.
Vitamin D	Fortified milk, liver, egg yolk, butter	Formed in the skin by exposure to ultraviolet light. Stored in liver. Large amounts are dangerous.
Vitamin E	Vegetable oils, green leafy vegetables, egg yolk	Large amounts can be harmful.
Vitamin K	Dark green leafy vegetables, cereals, egg yolk, milk	Synthesized by intestinal bacteria.

Source: Adapted from J. A. Eagles and M. N. Randall, *Handbook of Normal and Therapeutic Nutrition*. New York: Raven Press, copyright 1980. Used with permission.

hearts. There is no need for meat to be eliminated, but assisting patients to adjust even a few meals each week can significantly improve the dietary balance. Reductions in added salt and processed foods are also well-researched strategies for health promotion.

Supplements. As a general rule, patients should be counseled not to depend on vitamin and mineral supplements to meet their nutritional needs. Dependence on supplements reinforces the idea that individuals do not need to pay attention to or be concerned with what they are eating. Good nutrition goes far beyond the ingestion of vitamins and minerals to meet minimum daily requirements. Patients also need to be aware that it is possible to ingest too much of needed nutrients. Gastric irritation can result from excess ascorbic acid, and abnormal calcium deposits may occur from excess vitamin D.

Most of the essential vitamins and minerals are liberally distributed in foods, and meeting minimum daily requirements should not be difficult with a balanced diet. Calcium intake, however, may be deficient if an individual does not use milk products. Supplementation may then be appropriate for high-risk patients. Iron intake is also frequently deficient in typical American diets, and supplementation may be appropriate for anemic patients or those unwilling to include iron-rich foods in the diet. Additional supplementation is usually not necessary unless an individual is following a strict weight reduction regimen. Table 9-5 summarizes some basic data about essential vitamins and their rich sources in food.

Fatigue and Anorexia

Fatigue and anorexia can be serious problems for patients with rheumatoid arthritis and can significantly compromise the individual's overall nutritional status over the prolonged course of the disease. This is especially true for elderly patients and those who live alone.

Shopping and cooking for one can be a challenging and discouraging task when mealtimes are not accompanied by conversation or other social interaction. The effort to prepare food may not seem worth the price. Meal preparation needs to be included in the patient's overall plan for energy conservation and joint protection (see Chapter 3). The nurse can assist the patient to experiment with various adaptive aids, nutritious prepared foods, or external supports such as meals on wheels, which can help the patient meet nutritional needs in a nonstressful way.

The arthritis drug regimen can also complicate nutritional concerns, since gastric upset is such a frequent side effect of drug therapy. The nurse should reinforce teaching about the importance of buffering medications with food and fluid and should reassure the patient that gastric upset tends to lessen after a drug has been used for a few weeks. Special challenges will be presented by the use of oral corticosteroids, and major diet modifications may be required to counteract the common side effects of these drugs. Oral steroids profoundly influence metabolism even with short-term use, and can rapidly produce complications associated with sodium and water retention, weight gain, hyperglycemia, and protein catabolism.

Patients with mandibular involvement may have to face jaw pain and functional difficulties with chewing and swallowing as they attempt to eat. The nurse should assist patients to modify their meals so that they are low in volume and easily chewed, and yet maintain an adequate nutrient composition.

Chronic Inflammation

Frequent or prolonged episodes of inflammation may significantly alter a patient's protein and calorie requirements. Many factors affect energy requirements, but patients need to understand the basic relationships between inflammation and fever and increases in the basal metabolic rate. These concerns are particularly important for elderly patients. Where anorexia inhibits normal food intake, the patient's diet needs to be enriched with protein powders in milkshakes, puddings, and other such foods to maintain adequate body stores. Unless a patient is severely debilitated, a daily intake of 1.0–1.5 g of protein per kilogram of body weight should be sufficient to maintain a positive nitrogen balance.

Diet Therapy

Research to date has not supported the premise that any special foods or diet are of consistent benefit in improving the symptoms of arthritis or producing a cure. However, there are provocative study observations that seem to indicate that individualized diet therapy may be clinically useful in selected patients. The literature contains specific case reports of individual patients who have experienced significant improvement in symptoms while following an experimental diet. The idea of diet therapy is popular, as our society is programmed to blame various health problems on what we eat. The major problem, of course, is that variations in joint symptoms occur in arthritis patients on a day-to-day basis. It is therefore nearly impossible to accept or reject the effects of any specific diet changes.

Most experimental diets assume that certain foods act as noxious elements, producing the joint symptoms of rheumatoid arthritis as a form of hypersensitivity response. Most of these diets are therefore elimination diets that attempt to isolate and remove specific environmental food toxins. Sodium nitrates, black walnuts, dairy products, additives, alcohol, and red meat have all been targeted, either individually or in groups. Although this approach has been thoroughly disparaged by most treatment centers, current research on the immune response does indicate that diet may well influence inflammation. However, at this stage, the research is not complete enough to be translated into practical dietary guidelines for patients.

The nurse needs to be familiar with current developments in this area and act as a resource for patients and families. The patient should be encouraged to follow a sensible basic diet with the understanding that no known diet modification can predictably produce disease improvement. However, if a patient wishes to attempt diet modification and is in a good nutritional state, there is usually no reason for the nurse to argue against it. The nurse and patient can work together to analyze the proposed diet and ensure that the patient can meet nutritional needs within its restrictions. The patient should also be taught that when symptom improvements have occurred as an apparent result of diet changes, they appeared promptly, that is, within a few weeks. A restricted trial period of 6–10 weeks would therefore provide a reasonable time frame for evaluating the patient's response to the diet and should cause minimal disruption of the patient's total nutritional status. Continuation with the diet for a longer period is justified only if clinical improvement is seen, and then only in consultation with the physician.

Supporting patients in limited, controlled experimentation with diet therapy is very different from supporting patients who embrace food fads. Food faddism pervades daily American life and proliferates under free press and free speech constitutional guarantees. Food faddism is a multi-million-dollar industry that has been enthusiastically adopted by celebrities and businesses alike. Health books and other literature may be published and promoted without significant regard for accuracy and come under the jurisdiction of the Food and Drug Administration only if they are used in the direct sale of specific products.

It is difficult to enter a bookstore or pick up a magazine without encountering a new diet that claims to improve arthritis or reduce the risk of cancer. Knowing that they consume large amounts of processed foods, Americans are receptive to the myth that most if not all diseases are caused by faulty diet. Arthritis patients are particularly vulnerable because the control and relief provided by standard regimens is frequently inadequate.

The nurse needs to be aware of the scope of food faddism in arthritis and should help patients and families evaluate the various claims. Macrobiotic foods, alfalfa, yucca extract, aloe vera, seaweed, wheat germ, ginseng root, raw milk, fertile eggs, chinese herbs, and blackstrap molasses all have their supporters. The goal is to help the patient become a knowledgeable consumer and avoid the pitfalls of false advertising and inflated claims.

Nutrition and diet therapy are intriguing aspects of the home care management of arthritis. The nurse has multiple opportunities to increase the patient's knowledge about nutrition and assist in solving problems related to overweight or inadequate nutrition. Table 9-6 summarizes these basic strategies in a care plan format.

Table 9-6   Care Plan for Nutrition

Nursing Diagnosis	Patient Goal	Interventions
Altered nutrition: more than body requirements related to decreased activity and energy expenditure.	Patient will achieve a gradual weight loss of 1–2 pounds per week until desired weight is reached.	1. Explore patient's feelings concerning current weight and body image. 2. Reinforce teaching concerning the negative effects of excessive weight on joints. 3. Instruct patient on the relationship between activity and weight gain. 4. Teach the use of a daily food diary as a basis for diet analysis. 5. Establish a contract for weight loss and weight goals.
	Patient will modify dietary intake to match energy expenditure while maintaining a balanced diet.	1. Analyze patient's food diary and assist in developing strategies for calorie reduction and diet modification.

Table 9–6 Care Plan for Nutrition (*Cont.*)

Nursing Diagnosis	Patient Goal	Interventions
		2. Involve the family and social networks in the patient's effort to diet.
		3. Explore techniques for behavior modification of food habits.
		4. Refer patient to community weight reduction programs as appropriate.
	Patient will participate in frequent, regular exercise to tolerance.	1. Explore options for increasing daily energy expenditure without stressing the joints.
		2. Offer frequent monitoring, support, and encouragement for all efforts to diet.
		3. Encourage patient to become or remain active in family and social activities.
Altered nutrition: less than body requirements related to chronic pain, inflammation, fatigue, or anorexia.	Patient will eat a well-balanced, calorie-rich diet. Patient will restore or maintain weight in the desired range.	1. Assist patient to analyze daily food diary for the adequacy of total calories, protein, and other basic nutrients.
		2. Explore methods to enrich the current diet in needed directions.
		3. Suggest the use of small, frequent meals with supplements as indicated. Teach patient to avoid ingesting empty calories.
		4. Suggest vitamin/mineral supplements as indicated.
		5. Review joint protection and energy conservation strategies to ensure that the patient has adequate energy for meal preparation.

continued

Table 9–6   Care Plan for Nutrition (*Cont.*)

Nursing Diagnosis	Patient Goal	Interventions
		6. Suggest assistive devices as indicated for food preparation.
	Patient will adjust the diet appropriately to meet the demands of chronic inflammation or jaw pain.	1. Provide or reinforce teaching concerning the relationship of inflammation to body needs for protein and other nutrients. 2. Assist patient to adjust medication schedule as necessary to minimize gastric distress. 3. Involve the family and/or social networks in nutrition teaching. 4. Suggest strategies for enriching a soft or liquid diet during periods of jaw pain.

CASE STUDIES

1. Ben Jacobs is a 58-year-old retired man with osteoarthritis in his right hip that is significantly impairing his mobility. He has lived alone since the death of his wife last year and has no family in the immediate area. He has gained 35 pounds in the months since his wife's death and currently weighs 230 pounds on a 5 foot 10 inch large-boned frame.

    1. What assessment data would be appropriate to help you understand the scope of Mr. Jacobs' problems?
    2. What nutritional teaching might be appropriate?
    3. Mr. Jacobs desires to lose weight. What strategies could you suggest for helping him to alter his current dietary habits?
    4. What community supports might be helpful for Mr. Jacobs?

2. Esther Walker is a 48-year-old single woman who has had rheumatoid arthritis for 15 years. She has had increasing disease activity over the past 3 years and has

experienced several disease flare-ups, each of which persisted for several months. She has recently been started on penicillamine and is having significant gastric upset.

Ms. Walker is a thin, pale, frail-appearing woman who is experiencing chronic fatigue and pain in multiple joints. She admits to having very poor eating habits, as food has never been important to her. She dislikes cooking and lacks energy for food preparation. She never seems to have much of an appetite and says that she just seems to forget about shopping, cooking, and eating.

1. What additional assessment data would help you to understand the scope of Ms. Walker's nutritional problems?
2. What diet and nutrition teaching is needed?
3. What energy conservation principles might help Ms. Walker deal with the stresses of food preparation?
4. How can her diet be modified to better meet her ongoing nutritional needs?

PATIENT EDUCATION MATERIALS

Arthritis Foundation. (1982). *Diet and nutrition: Facts to consider.* Arthritis Foundation, Box 19000, Atlanta, GA 30326.

Halpern, A.A. (1984). Nutrition, arthritis and weight loss. In A.A. Halpern (ed.), *The Kalamazoo arthritis book.* George F. Stickley Co., 210 W. Washington Square, Philadelphia, PA 19106.

Hixson, C. (1977). *Arthritis food facts.* Arthritis Treatment Center, Rose Medical Center, 4567 E. 9th Ave., Denver, CO 80220.

BIBLIOGRAPHY

Eagles, J. A., & Randall, M. N. (1980). *Handbook of normal and therapeutic nutrition.* New York: Raven Press.

Greenwald, R. A. (1984). Lay literature dealing with dietary treatment of arthritis. *Clinical Rheumatology in Practice, 2*(3), 134–140.

Greenwald, R. A. (1986). Diet and arthritis: The myths and the facts. *Continuing Education for the Family Physician, 21*(2), 81–83.

Job, C., Menkes, C. J., & Delbarre, F. (1980). Zinc sulfate in the treatment of rheumatoid arthritis. *Arthritis and Rheumatism, 23,* 1408–1412.

Kowsari, B., Finnie, S. K., Carter, R. C., Love, J., Katz, P., Longley, S., & Panush, R. S. (1983). Assessment of the diet of patients with rheumatoid and osteoarthritis. *Journal of the American Dietetic Association*, *82*(6), 657–659.

Lorig, K., & Fries, J. F. (1980). *The arthritis helpbook*. Reading, Mass: Addison-Wesley.

Panush, R. S., Carter, R. L., Katz, L., Kowsari, B., Longley, S., & Finnie, S. (1983). Diet therapy for rheumatoid arthritis. *Arthritis and Rheumatism*, *26*(4), 462–471.

Panush R. S., & Endo L. P. (1986). Diet and unproven remedies. In W. Katz (ed.), *The diagnosis and management of rheumatic disease*, 2nd ed. (pp. 819–823). Philadelphia: J.B. Lippincott.

Panush, R. S. & Webster, E. M. (1986). In G. E. Ehrlich (ed.), *Rehabilitation and management of rheumatic conditions*, 2nd ed. (pp. 290–303) Baltimore: Williams & Wilkins.

Simkin, P. A. (1981). Treatment of rheumatoid arthritis with oral zinc sulfate. *Agents and Actions*, *8*, 587–589.

Webster, E. M., & Panush, R. S. (1984). Diet therapy for rheumatic disease. *Geriatric Medicine Today*, *3*(9), 61–63.

Ziff, M. (1983). Diet in the treatment of rheumatoid arthritis. *Arthritis and Rheumatism*, *26*(4), 457–461.

Index